Childhood Psychotherapy

Childhood Psychotherapy

A Bioenergetic Approach

Editor *Christa D. Ventling*, Basel

KARGER

Basel · Freiburg · Paris · London · New York ·
New Delhi · Bangkok · Singapore · Tokyo · Sydney

Christa D. Ventling, DPhil
Holbeinstrasse 65
CH-4051 Basel (Switzerland)

Library of Congress Cataloging-in-Publication Data

Childhood psychotherapy : a bioenergetic approach / editor, Christa D. Ventling.
p. cm.
Includes bibliographical references and indexes.
ISBN 3805571496 (hardcover : alk. paper)
1. Child psychotherapy. 2. Bioenergetic psychotherapy. 3. Psychoanalysis.
I. Ventling, Christa D.
[DNLM: 1. Psychotherapy--methods--Child. 2. Mind-Body Relations (Metaphysics)--Child. 3. Psychophysiology--Child. WS 350.2 C53635 2001]
RC489.B5 C48 2001
618.92′8914--dc21 00-048124

Drug Dosage. The authors and the publisher have exerted every effort to ensure that drug selection and dosage set forth in this text are in accord with current recommendations and practice at the time of publication. However, in view of ongoing research, changes in government regulations, and the constant flow of information relating to drug therapy and drug reactions, the reader is urged to check the package insert for each drug for any change in indications and dosage and for added warnings and precautions. This is particularly important when the recommended agent is a new and/or infrequently employed drug.

www.karger.com
Printed in Switzerland on acid-free paper by Reinhardt Druck, Basel
ISBN 3–8055–7149–6

Contents

Preface

This book is a unique addition to the flowering of research on infants and children. It is unique in that it focuses on the body experience of infants and children and utilisation of physical interventions in psychotherapy coming from clinical practice.

For years many of us have worked with the developmental arrests or early traumas in adults who have sought out bioenergetic analysis/therapy to help with their life problems. In this book we have represented some of those select few therapists who have treated these early problems before they have become fixed personality features or neurotic styles. The implications for *preventive treatment* are inspiring.

The book is meant to be practical and each chapter contains case histories or vignettes which illustrate the use of bioenergetic interventions. It is noteworthy that the interest in contributing to this volume came from members of the International Institute for Bioenergetic Analysis (IIBA) from a number of different countries on both sides of the Atlantic Ocean, underscoring the fact that this is a cross-cultural theme.

While genetic factors are continuing to be explored in laboratories of science, the data regarding aspects of nurture and relationship that impact the developing organism is provided from clinics, schools and consulting rooms. It is from this rich source that these writings have evolved. The pervasive influence of environment, the extent of parental ability to form attachment, and the quality of human interactions in the social sphere provide the ingredients that determine the developmental crucible of humanity for every person. This book represents a unique contribution to understanding the formation of the human being and what it means to be fully human.

William E. White, PhD
President, IIBA

Acknowledgements

This book would not exist today if I had not met Arnt Halsen in 1993. He planted the seed which eventually took shape and grew into this book. I am indebted to him for having opened my eyes and my mind to a different world than the one I knew then. Sadly and unexpectedly for all of us Arnt Halsen died in 1996. By reprinting his pioneering article here we pay him tribute.

It gives me great pleasure to acknowledge the co-operation of the contributing European and American authors. From the beginning, when there was only an idea and a call for papers, all of them were enthusiastic and motivated to share with me and our readers their personal experiences as psychotherapists.

During the more difficult times in the preparation of the manuscript I much depended upon the support of family, friends and colleagues. My deeply felt gratitude for their never-ending encouragement goes to my daughter Stephanie who followed my 9 months of 'writing-and-editing pregnancy' like a soul-mate with loving comments; to my son Derek who made me stick to the task by sending encouraging e-mails; to my friends, notably Ania Peter, who provided me with alarming historical anecdotes on child abuse, Vera Schenker, Sabine Sommer and Ursula Strebel, who 'mothered' me through, and last, but not least, to Lucas Carle, George Downing, Thomas Ehrensperger and Hugo Steinmann, professional colleagues, advisors and true friends. Finally, when the manuscript had turned into a book, I received excellent constructive criticism from Kai von Klitzing, for which I am much obliged.

I thank Anne Trager and Stephanie Ventling who have translated some of the articles into English, for their exceptional professionalism in both language and psychological terminology.

I feel honoured by the institutions who validated my efforts by granting me financial support. Thus I acknowledge with gratitude: my colleagues of the Swiss Society for Bioenergetic Analysis and Therapy (SGBAT), the European

Association for Body Psychotherapy, Switzerland (CH-EABP) and most of all the Uarda Frutiger Foundation of the Freiwillige Akademische Gesellschaft Basel (FAG) for their very generous contributions.

Finally, I thank Esther Bernhard, Angela Gasser, Anke Rogal and Rolf Steinebrunner of S. Karger AG Publishers who all shepherded me from editing to production with uninterrupted interest and patience and a singular human understanding.

Christa D. Ventling

August 2000

Ventling CD (ed): Childhood Psychotherapy. A Bioenergetic Approach.
Basel, Karger, 2001, pp 1–8

Introduction

Christa D. Ventling

A sandbox, dolls, puppets, figures representing animals and people, playhouses; materials for drawing, modelling and role-play – such is the traditional setting in psychoanalytical child therapies. The various playthings serve as projection objects for the child's feelings. The creative play represents a form of externalisation of inner, unconscious conflicts. The unanimated scenery becomes animated as these conflicts are made visible. The interpretations of the therapist help the child to recognise the type of relationship he has with his objects or art work. The transference is onto the therapist. The child is the choreographer in his own play and the therapist follows. He analyses the situation, and interacts verbally with the child on his level. When the therapeutic interpretations are addressing the unconscious fears of the child, for example, they can heal them indirectly [Kernberg, 2000].

Using bioenergetic techniques with children, the setting is not so very different. Here, instead of playing with toys or creating an art work, the physical body of the child, its structure and dynamics of moving and interacting with the therapist, form the basis for the projection of inner conflicts of the child. He is being observed and interacted with by the therapist who may use his own body feelings and reactions as physical countertransference [Clauer and Heinrich, 1999]. From bodily awareness and observation he can draw conclusions about the child's management of his conflicts. While play therapy with traumatised children has enjoyed a long tradition [von Klitzing et al., 2000], bioenergetic therapy with such children is new. In fact it is so new that we are still in the process of gathering case histories which, hopefully, some day will provide the basis for a theory.

This book, therefore, does not supply the reader with established concepts and their application to children. Rather, it is a first collection of explicit descriptions of clinical practice, aimed at pointing out new avenues and stimulating the curiosity of the readers. They are not 'recipes' to be simply copied but require a basic understanding of bioenergetic therapy and analysis (BAT). Therefore let us detour briefly into what BAT stands for.

BAT is a body-oriented form of psychotherapy which has its roots in classical psychoanalysis, e.g. it goes back to Freud and hence to Reich. Reich [1933] created the notion of 'character armoring' which he defined as the somatic expression a person withdraws into in response to the traumatising environment during development. This assumed relationship between body expression and neurosis was extensively studied by Lowen [1958] in years of systematic personal observations and descriptions of patients. He came to the conclusion that there exists a dialectical understanding of the relationship between body and mind. That understanding postulates that body and mind are a unity and that they can mutually influence each other. His observations carried him further to conclude that denying vital needs to a child during development will result in character structure problems which also find an expressional counterpart in the body. Movement and feelings are processes of the physical side of the body, thinking and images are functions of the mind. While in a healthy individual these functions are integrated and expressed with a sense of 'this is me', in a neurotic individual and even more so in psychotic states this integration is at fault. Consequently, such a person may carry an expression of his body and his face which does not at all correspond to the state of his true being. The famous 'Smile! and put up an appearance although you don't feel like it' is a mild and rather social form of a split between feeling and the expression of it. More serious is the suffering from chronic physical pain like in psychosomatic disorders.

One of the doctrines of bioenergetic thinking is '*that the body remembers even when the mind does not*'. According to this, traumatisations at a very early age would be stored in a physical, somatic form, since the mind is not sufficiently developed yet to deal with storing and recalling memories in a cognitive way. A baby or young child, who has been subjected to negligent or aggressive treatment, learns to minimize the suffering by adapting physically and closing up emotionally. Reich [1933] called this early survival mechanism 'armouring'. It is like the child would say: 'nobody will ever hurt me again as long as I stay this way'.

We are all familiar with the reaction of a child who faces an adult attacker about to hit the child or scream at him: the child pulls his arms up and tries to protect his face. We can easily imagine what will happen if such a child is constantly being harassed. He may develop, depending on his genetic mapping and his social surrounding, into a withdrawn and shy person or into a cold, ready-to-defend-himself adult. In both cases he split his true feeling – fear – off. It is not uncommon that the underlying fear – in this case – may find a somatic outlet later in adult life [Ehrensperger, 1991].

Since its beginning with Lowen [1958, 1975], BAT was developed further both in theory and techniques by students and followers, especially those of the present second (and third) generation [Büntig, 1983; Geissler, 1994; Johnson, 1994; to name just a few]. Other body therapists have also made important contributions [Keleman, 1985; Boadella, 1991; Downing, 1994]. The techniques in BAT are interventions on a physical level during the context of a therapeutic session. These can encompass the entire range from just a gesture or a holding of the eye contact, for example, to a cathartic expression of an emotion by the patient. These bodily expressions usually lead to a new body consciousness and/or new insights, which the patient with the help of the therapist integrates into his own history. Lowen [1975] and his followers created many such interventions for specific situations, problems or character styles. The underlying concept (Lowen speaks about somatic blockages or blockages of energy flow) is to make the body more energetic, to bring life back into the body, hence the term bioenergetic. If we remember the term 'character-armour' such an approach makes sense.

An example of one of the key 'exercises' (this terminology in my mind is not a good one as it could mislead the reader into thinking that the interventions in BAT are merely gymnastic exercises – which they are not) is the following called 'grounding': the feet are firmly planted, even pushed into the ground, the effort of which will invariably be felt as an awareness of one's own body. It is a stress position which through the simple effort of maintaining it for a while will increase the breathing and sensitize the person to existing tensions in his body. From the position of being firmly grounded, the patient may be able to suddenly loosen up a certain tension inside the body and have an emotional outbreak or generate a new insight into a problem.

Many such exercises or interventions are available for work with adult patients. The idea that one could modify the techniques and adapt them to children probably first occurred to Arnt Halsen. In 1993 he presented his bioenergetic approach in working with very young physically abused children at a European workshop. He explained how he had modified certain basic 'exercises' of Lowen originally designed to increase bodily consciousness and physical awareness to suit children. He illustrated his theoretical concepts with individual case histories. I was impressed with what he had achieved given the severity of these traumatised children. I also sensed that Halsen had reported a pilot project with a future. The general audience, however, was not especially impressed and did not pay him the tribute he deserved. Later a discouraged Halsen shared with me his deeply felt wish for a more understanding professional world. We discussed ways of making bioenergetic psychotherapy for traumatised children a real issue and how to raise interest among our professional societies. A call for an informal get-together of interested colleagues in Switzerland failed, but during a Conference of Bioenergetics in Arles in 1997, a few colleagues signalled various degrees of interest. The idea of collecting articles came up and I enthusiastically wrote to Halsen about the plans. It was a bolt from the blue to learn that my letter found no destination as Arnt Halsen had passed away the year before. The incentive to create a book prevailed, however, and I also saw it as a way to give Arnt Halsen the recognition he did not get during his lifetime. I got in touch with his widow about my plans and she supported me gratefully. My call for papers found an echo. The time seemed right to bring bioenergetic techniques adapted to working with children to the general audience of child psychotherapists. I was very happy about this.

What possible traumas are we dealing with in young children and what bodily interventions seem suitable with them?

Let us have a look first at the mothers-to-be and their possible problems with the notion that they are going to be shortly with a baby. Those who find their way into therapy do have serious worries. It could be that they never wanted this pregnancy and are emotionally 'at war' with the developing foetus. It could be that their economic situation seems so hopeless that they become self-destructive, e.g. through drugs, and as a consequence worry even more about the health of the child, a vicious circle. Or the possibility of a genetic disorder robs them their peace of mind. Or like a patient of mine who had just worked up the courage to sue for a divorce from her abusing husband and found herself pregnant. All these women are deeply unhappy and the fears or the self-destruction are often increasing almost exponentially towards the end of the pregnancy. Unless we therapists manage to ready such a woman for accepting her child, the baby is facing a first trauma: rejection. Often the women are torn between feelings of love and hate for the baby or despair and guilt. The forthcoming birth may bring up fears of not being able to cope and not being able to properly take care of the child. In the chapter on Birth and Bonding, I am describing a bioenergetic sensitising technique which is meant to increase awareness and perception in the mother-to-be as a preparation to a better 'reading' and understanding of the needs of the baby. The effect of the exercise usually is that it raises curiosity about the competence of the baby they are carrying. This is often the beginning of a caring relationship. A realistic account of therapy with a mother-to-be and the quality of her relationship with her unborn child is provided by *Vincentia Schroeter*.

There exists vast literature on the problems of early separation, the subsequent lack of trust due to a non-existent or bad-quality bonding and the problem of not being able to form lasting relationships. Separation from the caretaker will invariably have an impact on the character structure of the child.

As adults these persons often display signs of anxiously avoiding relationships which is first of all mirrored in the therapeutic setting. The fact that after a successful therapy they are able to enter relationships shows that this particular problem has good healing chances.

There are many reasons for a separation of mother and child following birth and many of them unwanted by the mother. A new-born infant may be denied the close contact with his mother/caretaker for the reason that he required intensive medical care due to some medical problem after birth. It prevented the mother/caretaker from being with the child. Since a new-born infant has no notion of time, once the wish to be close is there, any length of time away from the mother equals an eternity. Here we are encountering a first separation trauma. If the infant cannot assimilate this experience it will withdraw emotionally and later develop a distrusting attitude. Denial of a symbiotic relationship with his mother/caretaker is a serious trauma for a baby. When such a baby is a toddler or even older, he will often display a very demanding regressive or a very distanced behaviour. Mothers are often at a loss. *Jens Kühntopp* and *Vita Heinrich* have performed the task to develop certain bioenergetic interventions for mother-child dyads that diagnostically measure the quality of the relationship. They provide a moving account of 2 cases and the consequences of the diagnosis.

Some children are born into this world already afflicted with problems. Twenty years ago the statistics (in Germany) stated that 30–80% of all children born had one or several problems as the postnatal examination revealed. This percentage has now decreased, but even 30% are still too high. This places enormous demands on the caretakers, who usually is the mother. The child may be born with an unrecognised or undiagnosed deficit which appears only years later in conjunction with social interactions. The postnatal and early childhood development may be hindered or slowed down or follow an unusual path. Hyperactivity or a psycho-organic syndrome (POS) is seemingly more common nowadays. *Tom Wills*, a child psychotherapist originally from the behavioural school, has successfully tried to integrate some of Halsen's exercises into the sessions with severely disturbed and/or hyperactive hospitalised children and gives a detailed account of some cases.

The painful experiences babies and small children endure and the mechanisms and forms of survival have many different facets. Separation from their mothers at birth or at any time thereafter is a major trauma, but no experience is as devastating to body and soul as physical and sexual abuse. These children show severe behavioural problems and are extremely difficult to work with. The report of *Arnt Halsen* tells us about his experiences with such hospitalised children and gives a moving account of how much energy and diligent daily work is needed to re-establish trust in these young children.

Separation and neglect of babies always have serious consequences, but so has the opposite, e.g. overstimulation. Babies normally have a very well-developed sense of when enough is enough and this already from birth. For example, when they have enough to drink, they turn their head away from the source or go to sleep. When they do not like what is happening, they scream. It happens that some babies are not allowed to be on their own and whenever awake receive too much attention of the wrong kind. They end up being overstimulated by their caretakers and must withdraw emotionally for their own protection. Here, any bioenergetic exercise or intervention would have to be extremely carefully considered first in order to rule out another overstimulation. *Suzanne B. Robert-Ouvray*, an analytically trained and extremely sensitive child therapist, carried out a long and difficult therapy with an overstimulated child and explains the theory behind her treatment.

A single overwhelming experience can produce a shock, a repetition of this event will reproduce the emotional state of the first time. Adaptation to everyday life is most likely characterised by some highly individual (often socially contraproductive) behaviour as survival mechanisms – which we call post-traumatic stress syndrome (PTSS). What does this mean on a psychobiological level? The crucial psychological process here is dissociation. It means that the intense emotions associated with the traumatic experience caused memories to be dissociated from consciousness and to be stored as we now know in a somatic memory [van der Kolk, 1994; van der Kolk and Fisler, 1995]. The hypothalamic-pituitary-adrenal axis, a finely tuned system producing several hormones influencing each other, is the key to understanding the emotional state of human beings [Pert, 1997]. Important for us therapists to remember is that posttraumatic reactions, like the original traumatic reactions, are biologically encoded. A spontaneous recovery is not possible. A literature search for treatment models reveals that most do not take the physiological side sufficiently into account and preferentially support cognitive-behavioural frameworks [Eagle, 1998; Wilson et al., 1995]. These involve telling/re-telling the story, sometimes with the help of guided imagery [Singer, 1974], normalising the symptoms, addressing guilt feelings and encouraging mastery, all within the protective therapeutic setting and the demonstrated ability of the therapist to tolerate the overwhelming aspects of the trauma. While this approach may be successful to a certain degree with adult patients, it will fail with children below the age of logical thinking. To differentiate fantasy from reality is not possible for children younger than approximately 7 years of age. The younger they were when the trauma occurred, the greater will be the amnesia which followed the devastating fear of being killed or the agony over extreme physical pain. The undeniable and in the meantime proven physiological substrate [van der Kolk et al., 1996] in modern body-oriented psychotherapy is being taken into account. Here may be our chance when working with traumatised children.

While Pierre Janet [1925, cited in van der Kolk and van der Hart, 1989] is credited to have been the first to study systematically dissociation as a result of shock trauma, Levine [1990, 1997] and van der Kolk [1994] and van der Kolk et al. [1996] must be mentioned for their innovative therapeutic approaches. Basically their methods are based on a re-en-activation of *both the lost memory* in conjunction with the *emotional state* of the moment of the traumatic experience in the protected setting of the therapeutic practice. It is virtually a reversal of the original 'going numb' on all levels, a reversal of the physiological reactions from hence. It is not an easy technique with adults and usually requires long-term therapy. There are no reports as yet to our knowledge on how the technique should be used on very young children. Therefore, I must give credit to *Rainer Mahr* for his courage to try this method on 2 young patients who suffered profound traumas from separation and war experiences.

This manual is a modest, albeit first effort, to bring to a wider public the techniques of bioenergetic therapy adapted to treat traumatised children. The authors of this book make no claim that their techniques should replace the traditional method of analytical play-therapy. They hope, however, that BAT could be accepted as an alternative and/or additional method to child psychotherapy and thus provide an enrichment to the prevailing classical child psychotherapy. They also hope to find colleagues who will be sufficiently intrigued by the perspectives offered to become motivated to learn and use some of the techniques on their young patients.

References

Boadella D (1991) Befreite Lebensenergie. Einführung in die Biosynthese. Kösel, München.

Büntig WE (1983) Bioenergetik; in Corsini RJ (Hrsg): Handbuch der Psychotherapie. Belz, Weinheim/Basel.

Clauer J, Heinrich V (1999) Körperpsychotherapeutische Ansätze in der Behandlung traumatisierter Patienten: Körper, Trauma und Seelenlandschaften. Zwischen Berührung und Abstinenz. Psychother Forum 7:75–93.

Downing G (1994) The Body and the Word. Routledge, New York. (In German: Körper und Wort in der Psychotherapie. Kösel, München 1996.)

Eagle GT (1998) An integrative model for brief term intervention in the treatment of psychological trauma. Int J Psychother 3:135–146.

Ehrensperger T (1991) Psychosomatische Medizin und bioenergetische Analyse; in Hoffmann-Axthelm D (Hrsg): Der Körper in der Psychotherapie. Transform, Oldenburg, pp 156–178.

Geissler P (1994) Psychoanalyse und Bioenergetische Analyse. Lang, Frankfurt.

Johnson SM (1994) Character Styles. Norton, New York.

Keleman S (1985) Emotional Anatomy. Center Press, Berkeley.

Kernberg PF (2000) The Forms of Play; in von Klitzing K, Tyson P, Bürgin D (eds): Psychoanalysis in Childhood and Adolescence. Karger, Basel, pp 25–41.

Levine P (1990) Der Körper als Heiler. Energie Charakter 2:22–43.
Levine P (1997) Waking the Tiger: Healing Trauma. North Atlantic Books, Berkeley.
Lowen A (1958) The Physical Dynamics of Character Structure. Grune & Stratton, New York. (In German: Körperausdruck und Persönlichkeit. Kösel, München 1980.)
Lowen A (1975) Bioenergetics. (In German: Bio-Energetik – Therapie der Seele durch Arbeit mit dem Körper. Rowohlt, Reinbek 1988.)
Pert CB (1997) Molecules of Emotion. Simon & Schuster; London.
Reich W (1933) Charakteranalyse (reprinted: Kiepenheuer & Witsch, Köln 1989).
Singer J (1974) Imagery and Day Dream Methods in Psychotherapy and Behaviour Modification. Academic Press, New York.
van der Kolk BA, van der Hart O (1989) Pierre Janet and the Breakdown of Adaptation in Psychological Trauma. Am J Psychiatry 146:1530–1540.
van der Kolk BA (1994) The Body Keeps the Score: Memory and the Evolving Psychobiology of Posttraumatic Stress. Harv Rev Psychiatry 1:253–265.
van der Kolk BA, Fisler R (1995) Dissociation and the fragmentary nature of traumatic memories: Overview and exploratory study. J Trauma Stress 8:505–526.
van der Kolk BA, McFarlane A, van der Hart O (1996) A general appoach to treatment of post-traumatic stress disorder; in van der Kolk BA, McFarlane A, Waisaeth L (eds): Traumatic Stress: The Effect of Overwhelming Experience on Mind, Body and Society. Guilford Press, New York.
von Klitzing K, Tyson P, Bürgin D (eds) (2000) Psychoanalysis in Childhood and Adolescence. Karger, Basel.
Wilson SA, Becker LE, Tinker RH (1995) Eye movement desensitisation and reprocessing (EMDR) treatment for psychologically traumatised individuals. J Consult Clin Psychol 63:928–937.

Ventling, Christa D. (1930), 2 children, 3 grandchildren, studied chemistry at the University of Lausanne, Switzerland, and biochemistry at the University of Oxford, where she obtained a DPhil in 1957. After being active in medically oriented scientific research for many years she took up the study of psychology at the University of Basel, Switzerland, where she graduated in 1987. She worked in a psychiatric out-patient clinic before starting on her own as a psychotherapist. By 1995 she had completed her training as a bioenergetic therapist. Her main interest focuses on neuropsychobiology and unaltered from the time she was active in biochemical research, the origin of matter. She lives near Basel, Switzerland, where she has a private practice. She is a member of the editorial board of *Bioenergetic Analysis.*

Dr. phil. Christa D. Ventling, Holbeinstrasse 65, CH–4051 Basel (Switzerland)

Ventling CD (ed): Childhood Psychotherapy. A Bioenergetic Approach.
Basel, Karger, 2001, pp 9–18

Birth and Bonding: To Be or Not To Be

Christa D. Ventling

A baby is born.

A small human being equipped with the bare essentials to make himself heard, to grasp for a warm skin to attach, to find a nipple to drink from, a baby totally dependent on a mother for physical and emotional survival. A baby in search of a bond. Bonding means survival. Not bonding means doom. It is truly an issue of life or death.

Historical Atrocities and Early Insights

The Emperor Frederick II (1194–1250) of Hohenstaufen was probably the first person in history to test in a scientific way the life-or-death issue of the mother-infant relationship. Actually, this was not what he meant to explore. Rather, he wanted to find out whether the acquirement of language in infants occurred by learning from others or through innate knowledge. For this purpose, he forbade the nurses of an orphanage to ever speak to the infants. The shocking result was that all these infants, in spite of being fed and looked after, died [Christoffel, 1965]. The conclusions that the Emperor drew from this are unknown to us, but we must assume that besides the lack of verbal communication something else very basic to life was missing. In this century much evidence about the long-term neurotisising effect of what we now call hospitalism, the syndrome which consists of depression, withdrawal, apathy, even retardation and more, has been obtained. Durfee and Wolf [1934], Lowrey [1940], Bender and Yarnell [1941], Bakwin [1942], Goldfarb [1944], Spitz [1945, 1946a, 1946b, 1950], Bowlby [1951] and Dührssen [1958], all published investigations about traumatising effects in children brought up in institutions. An 8-month-long hospitalisation of small children resulted in very grave psychopathological effects [Durfee and Wolf, 1934] and a 3-year institutionalisation [Lowrey, 1940; Bender and Yarnell,

1941; Goldfarb, 1944] produced irreversible damage. Spitz's [1945, 1946, 1950] investigations are probably the best known. He studied 21 children of an institution during 2 years and found them severely retarded with regard to language comprehension and muscular skills. In another report he describes 34 children who, after a period of up to 6 months after birth with their mothers, were placed in an institution. There, some affective contact with the nurses was possible, yet, proportional to the duration of the separation from their mothers these children developed disturbances which Spitz called 'anaclitic depression'. The children became lethargic, refused to eat, made no sounds anymore and many eventually died like a candle going out. Spitz was probably first at pointing out the absolute necessity of regular and maintained physical, sensual and emotional contact between the mothering person and the child for the formation of a life-sustaining relationship. In his study all of this was not possible because of the shortage of caretakers in relation to the large number of babies. Dührssen [1958] confirmed Spitz's observations when reporting his comparative investigation of children in institutions, in foster families and in their original families. The children living their early life in the original homes had far fewer behavioural problems and were far more advanced in their social competence. The crowning evidence for the importance of loving physical contact between mother and child, however, came years later when Harlow and Suomi [1974] showed that the substitution of a real monkey mother by a wire-surrogate made the baby monkey apathetic and depressed.

Bonding Issues and Developmental Consequences

Whatever the social interaction pattern later in life will be, the prototype is established in the first 6 months [Stern, 1953]. During this time period the infant has learnt how to get his mother to respond to his signals, how to play with him, how to maintain the flow of social exchanges, and how and which signals to use in order to stop or to avoid an unwanted situation. Thus, we know now that the causes for adult neurotic or psychotic behaviour problems date much further back than the oedipal age of 4–5 years as Sigmund Freud had made us believe. The earliest period immediately after birth is indeed crucial, and so are the first 2 years of life, the preverbal period, where the baby must use body language together with vocal sounds in order to be understood and to have his needs satisfied. The baby will try very hard, but even a baby has his limits. The attachment of the baby to his mother is not only significant, but absolutely necessary [Bowlby, 1969]. Children who are separated from their mothers develop a deep longing to the original attachment situation. The longing can be so intense that the children fall into a state of pathological grief. Bowlby draws the conclusion that the loss of a partner later in life can then reproduce a similar pathological condition. Clearly disturbances due to separation of even short duration of the newly born infant from his mother can have serious consequences later in life. The quality of the attachment predicts the quality of the exploration of 1-year-olds: those with a good attachment are more daring, more curious, more adventuresome in a strange situation, they let their mothers go, feel secure in exploring the room, even when they lose eye contact and return to her. Those with one form of insecure attachment (several forms are described) would cling longer, feel anxious in a new situation and let their mothers go only for short moments [Ainsworth and Bell, 1970]. It seems paradoxical, but the child who had a firm and trustworthy attachment can let go easier than a child whose attachment was rather week or ambivalent.

Baby or Mother: Who Bonds Whom?

We may be inclined to think that bonding starts with birth, but there is evidence that it may in fact start much sooner, much before birth, weeks before the mother and the baby have looked into each others eyes. Sometime after the 16th week of pregnancy the mother can feel the faint movements of the foetus who is no more than 18 cm long. Interviews with mothers invariably reveal how they long for this moment. When it finally happens and they sense these movements like wings of a butterfly flapping they are moved in awe. They feel a deep love emerging. This is *prenatal* bonding. We also speak about prenatal bonding injury: this occurs when the baby is unwanted and not communicated with. Pre- and perinatal research seems to support this. Verny [1993] showed that the foetus has a life of its own and at birth already a history – though short – of its own [Chamberlain, 1994].

The modern technique of analysing video films in slowed down motion [Stern, 1997] have provided us with hitherto unavailable evidence to understand how perinatal bonding is established. The early thinking that the mothers or caretakers initiate the subsequent bonding is no longer valid – it is the baby who sends out signals in form of sensomotoric expressions to which the mother responds. He enters her into a dialogue absolutely necessary as stimulation for optimum physical and psychological growth. It is the beginning of a continued interaction with repeats and new signals between mother and child which finally forms and firmly establishes what we call bonding. Stern [1997] also speaks about a 'dance' between mother and child.

Encouraging Bonding

In the 1950s, after Spitz had published his dramatic findings about the orphanage children, paediatricians, obstetricians, nurses and psychiatrists became slowly more aware about the damaging effects of separation of infants from their mothers. But in those years it was still customary for a mother to labour alone and to deliver a baby in the absolute sterility of the operating room and to be separated from her baby thereafter for some hours; bottle feeding was favoured over breast-feeding. Most people accepted these conditions without questioning. A few, however, started to doubt whether such a procedure would be beneficial to the physical and emotional health of both mother and child. Clearly history had provided sufficient evidence about the damaging effect of separation of mother and child and about the damaging effect of lack of handling the children. The importance of attachment, of forming a bond between mother and child, as Bowlby's [1969] work had shown, could no longer be ignored. All these issues became crucial for premature infants who must be placed in incubators with life-sustaining and -saving machines. They are already at high risk for genetic or birth process reasons. Their perception of the outside world takes place through glass or plastic walls. The monotonous humming of the life-sustaining machines is anything else but an auditory stimulation. All of this and the lack of interaction with a loving human being, or of feeling the warm touch accompanied by the soothing voice of the mother, are severe risks for a normal development of the child. Klaus and Kennel [1970] were probably the first to implicate special sensory stimulation programmes in order to overcome the isolation and deadening sounds of the machines surrounding the premature infants. Ruth Rice [1979] introduced what became known as the therapeutic touch [see also Montague, 1971]. This programme consisted of a combination of touch or gentle massage and rocking along with auditory and visual stimulation which the mothers of the premature infants administered four times a day during 1 month. When these infants, together with the (untreated) controls, were examined 4 months later, the treated infants showed significant gains in neurological and mental development and weight compared to the non-treated infants. Candice Pert [1987] offers an explanation: tactile stimulation of an infant such as massage of loving touch and stroking the spinal column should have the effect of stimulating the 'nodal points'. These are specific places on the body where there are high concentrations of neuropeptides which are activated and send messages to the hypothalamus and immune system, which in turn would stimulate and activate healing processes, stimulate weight gain, regulate sleep and respiratory processes. Klaus and Kennel [1977] showed that babies who were allowed to remain with their mothers for the first few hours after birth were better off psychologically 5 years later than those babies who had been separated right away. They advocated that mothers and their full-term infants not be separated for reasons of the essential bonding.

With the introduction of Leboyer's [1986] concept of natural childbirth in the 1970s, a movement started whereby one suddenly remembered old cultural customs and techniques around childbirth. These were notably two: the older, wiser women who assist young women in childbirth, and the intimate physical contact through loving strokes which mother hands perform on the body of their new-born babies.

In the 1970s, Klaus and Kennel studied the advantages of mothering the mothers, as they called it, by having a 'doula' present during labour and childbirth. A doula (greek: douleia, meaning originally slave work) is an experienced woman who helps other women in childbirth by providing continuous physical, emotional and informational support before, during and after childbirth. Klaus et al. [1993] carried out controlled studies in Houston and Guatemala, and for a number of parameters they documented scientifically the beneficial effects of doula support during labour and birth. The data are impressive: the presence of a doula reduced the overall caesarean section rate by 50%, length of labour by 25%, oxytocin use by 40%, pain medication by 30%, the need for forceps by 40% and requests for epidurals by 60%. The doula group mothers also said they spent less time away from their babies, and it took them an average of 2.9 versus 9.8 days for the non-doula group to develop a relationship with their babies. These results suggest that support during labour expedited the doula group mothers' readiness to fall in love with their babies and that this attachment made them less willing to be away from them.

In the 1950s, Wilhelm Reich disclosed his ideas about prevention of traumatic experiences very early in life which he saw as potential seeds for later chronic depression, schizophrenia and antisocial behaviour [Reich, 1933, 1951]. His vision was intensive care and support of women in pregnancy, support during labour and the weeks after the birth, diagnosis and prevention of armouring and long-term studies thereafter of such children; however, his vision never materialised. His daughter Eva Reich, influenced by his thinking, developed, partly influenced by Leboyer and others, what became known in the 1970s as 'Gentle Bioenergetics', a supportive therapeutic concept for women before, during and after childbirth. It includes a special type of baby massage, done by the mother to her baby.

Now infant massages or stroking is being practised in many cultures and is based on a very long tradition. Indian, as well as African and Caribbean women and many others, regularly use nut oil to massage their babies' skin and spend time doing loving strokes and passive movements on their babies' joints. Leboyer [1986], deeply impressed, brought this loving technique from India in the 1970s.The tactile stimulation is supposed to have a positive influence on myelination of the central nervous system [Rice, 1979]. Both babies and mothers appear to gain great pleasure and comfort from these activities. With this close physical relationship there comes also a great deal of emotional contentment and well-being. Eva Reich named her baby massage 'Butterfly Massage' because the warm hand or fingers of the mother move tenderly over the skin of the baby with just enough pressure to assure a good contact. The mother stays also in eye contact with the baby and she speaks to him in a soft loving voice. The child receives an optimum stimulation of all his senses. This creates a feeling of wellness in the baby. Sometimes the stimulation of the nerve endings in the skin causing a tender vibration allows the baby to go deeper into contact with the mother and establish the bond. According to Eva Reich this is what prevents armouring, and this is what can heal a poor-quality bonding between mother and child. She considers bonding a bioenergetic process. She has taught this for most of her life with great success [Reich and Zornanszky, 1997] (For other excellently illustrated guide books on baby massage see also Leboyer [1986], Walker [1995] and Velten and Walter [1997]). An impressive account of a new-born healed with her method is recalled by Wendelstadt [1998].

Enter the Therapist

Bonding creates a feeling of safety, a place from which to experience the world, a place of security and confidence, bonding means love. A good bonding is the key for a happy and healthy child, and the world will appear friendly to him. If bonding does not happen or is unreliable, then the rest of the world becomes a mirror image, a frightening unknown world. Lack of bonding – as we know now – occurs through lack of skin contact, lack of sensual stimulation. We assume that this most likely leads to a shutting down of the development of the emotional (right) hemisphere of the brain in favour of the thinking (left) hemisphere. In other words, this could be the beginning of the mind/body split. Poorly bonded babies will grow into insecure adults, driven to figure out how to get by, how to cope and how to control situations. They live their life from their heads and prefer to ignore their emotional centre, which could throw them out of control [Rand, 1996]. What can we as therapists do? Can we really influence the vital bonding? Yes, we can. I believe that with a pregnant woman as a client we therapists have a twofold task. As a patient no doubt she deserves help. But, this patient does not come alone into therapy, she is carrying a baby and we are constantly aware of this. The foetus/baby enters the therapy as well, though unseen, and we can feel his presence. As therapists I believe we also have a moral obligation to educate her about the necessity of bonding. It may be the rare therapeutic situation when educating the client is part of the therapy.

(1) We can encourage and support the *prenatal bonding*. Often clients bring along the first ultrasound photograph and feel very excited about it but also very insecure. They may be overwhelmed by feelings of awe, of doubt, of pleasure, of fear before the unknown and everything at the same time. They need our empathy and our support. It is almost as if they would regress themselves into a state of helplessness and dependency. What they need is a therapeutic 'parenting', a sort of therapeutic form of 'mothering the mother'. Body psychotherapists are especially qualified here. We can be witness to movements of the baby and the mother's feelings about it. The loving touch starts with the mothers.

(2) We can teach them why it is important that they ask for delivery conditions which guarantee that their baby will not be taken away, be it only for a few hours. We can make them aware that the most dramatic trauma for a new-born is separation from the mother. We can point out to them the dreadful loneliness the baby finds himself in. For the baby who has no sense of time any separation is too long to bear. The threat of never being together again with the mother is omnipresent and is equivalent to dying. The defence of the newly born against such a terrible fate is emotional withdrawal. This seriously threatens the bonding. Many forms of depression later in life can be traced back to the earliest time of life, to the context of a deficient primary relationship.

(3) We can do certain exercises with them which increase their perception and their confidence in being able to 'read' the baby after birth. But, let us first look at the sensory development status of a new-born. The olfactory, tactile, auditory and visual senses develop prior to birth and reach a degree which we can compare to a 'starter kit' for the new-born to enable him to make contact and respond to it. The great pioneer Piaget [1950, 1959] perceived and minutely studied these senses and their further development in 2 of his own children from birth to 2 years. Piaget attentively followed every single movement, recorded and interpreted it in great detail, with all their repeats and variations on the theme. At first these senses were not in concert, the baby would touch or grab something and let go and repeat this, while looking somewhere else, but eventually the baby learnt for example to look first at the object before grabbing it. The tactile sense was from now on directed. From these sensomotoric explorations, coupled with active visual or auditory participation, Piaget constructed his theory of how intelligence is being built. Piaget had an extraordinary gift of perception, a scientific mind and a delightful

writing style. We bioenergetic therapists could almost call it 'body reading of the baby'. Starting from there, we can help the pregnant woman improve her own perceptiveness in order to understand and relate better to her baby. For this purpose I do passive awareness exercises. They are well received by patients and considered very helpful. They are non-verbal, silent exercises, I give directions, but after that we are perfectly quiet. As a start, I ask the client to find a comfortable position, to relax, maybe to place her hands over her belly and breathe normally.

Awareness of Shape. After a moment of quietness I ask her to let her eyes wander about the room, even out of the window and to note in her mind everything which is round, for example. She should then close her eyes and repeat the 'walk' around the room. When done she should open her eyes again as a signal to me. I then ask her to tell me what she noticed and sort of repeat the 'walk' with her. Clients are often shocked to find that they speak about a certain object as being round, because they *know* it is round, but from the angle where they are sitting the object appears oval, not round. They learn the difference between perceiving and knowing or believing of seeing correctly quite quickly. In another session such an exercise can be done with square instead of round objects, for example. It is advisable to do no more than one exercise of this kind in each session. This way the client often goes home and practices on the way!

Awareness of Colour. This exercise is done like the one above about shape, only this time the client must note in her mind everything which is of a given colour, e.g. red. A good idea is to choose a colour which is NOT predominant in the room.

Awareness of Noise. For this exercise it is not necessary to have a soundproof practice, on the contrary. The client is asked to notice anything she hears with open eyes first and then with closed eyes. This exercise should be done for 5 min. Noises can be in the room or coming from the outside or from inside the client's belly. The surprise here is usually the difference of perceiving noises with closed eyes versus open eyes.

Awareness of Odour. This is not really a passive exercise. I ask the client while still sitting, to start out by recording the smell of the room, through deep breathing, with eyes closed and also open, to note a possible difference. Does it remind her of something? I then ask her to walk around the room and feel free to put her nose to the furniture, the desktop, the window or the rug, for example, again with and without eyes closed, sniffing and recording. Finally I ask her to smell her own skin on her arms, her hands, maybe her hair. They are usually amazed how many different odours there are!

The new-born can differentiate sour smell from sweet smell and his preference for the sweet smell will guide him to find the nipple on his mother's breast which delivers the deliciously sweet milk, that his hands can touch, grasp and discriminate between cloth or the mother's skin, that he can turn his head to the direction from where he hears his name being called by his mother or other sounds, that he relaxes when being touched by his mother (or father's) hands and he can clearly look into the eyes of his mother and 'take her in' when she holds him in her arms. These facts become so much more meaningful after having gone through these exercises, the mothers tell me.

Perception exercises tend to bring our pregnant clients to a greater sensitivity and awareness to the sounds and reactions of the baby. We can relate to them the importance of physical contact, of tender loving touch. I firmly believe that by doing this their self-confidence as mothers is increased and they will apply their own responses to the baby in subtle and sensitive ways.

References

Ainsworth MDS, Bell SM (1970) Attachment, exploration and separation: Illustrated by the behavior of one-year-olds in a strange situation. Child Dev 41:49–67.

Bakwin H (1942) Loneliness in Infants. Am J Dis Child 63:30.

Bender L, Yarnell H (1941) An Observation Nursery: A Study of 250 Children in the Psychiatric Division of Bellevue Hospital. Am J Psychiatry 97:1158.

Bowlby J (1951) Maternal Care and Mental Health. Bull Ment Health Organ 3:355.

Bowlby J (1969) Attachment and Loss, vol. 1: Attachment. Basic Books, New York.

Chamberlain D (1994) How pre-and perinatal psychology can transform the world. Pre- Perinat Psychol J 8: 187–199.

Christoffel H (1965) Skizzen zur menschlichen Entwicklungspsychologie, Klett, Stuttgart.

Dührssen A (1958) Heimkinder und Pflegekinder in ihrer Entwicklung. Verlag für Medizinische Psychologie, Göttingen.

Durfee H, Wolff K (1934) Anstaltspflege und Entwicklung im ersten Lebensjahr. Z Kinderforsch 42:273.

Goldfarb W (1944) Effects of Early Institutional Care on Adolescent Personality: Rorschach Data. Am J Orthopsychiatry 14:441.

Goldfarb W (1947) Variations in adolescent adjustment of institution-reared children. Am J Orthopsychiatry 17:449.

Harlow HF, Suomi SJ (1974) Induced Depression in Monkeys. Behav Biol 12:273–296.

Klaus MH, Kennel JH (1970) Mothers separated from their newborn infants. Pediatr Clin North Am 17:1015–1037.

Klaus M, Kennel JH (1977) Impact of early separation and loss on family development: Maternal-infant-bonding. Mosby, St. Louis.

Klaus MH, Kennel JH, Klaus PH (1993) Mothering the Mother. Perseus Books, Reading.

Leboyer F (1986) Sanfte Hände. Kösel; München (original Gentle Hands, the Traditional Art of Indian Baby Massage, 1979).

Lowrey LG (1940) Personality distortion and early institutional care. Am J Orthopsychiatry 10:576.

Montague A (1971) Touching: The Human Significance of the Skin. Columbia University Press, New York.

Pert CB (1987) Neuropeptides. The emotions and bodymind. Noetic Sci Rev 2:13–18.

Pert CB (1997) Molecules of Emotion. Simon & Schuster, London.

Piaget J (1950) La construction du réel chez l'enfant. Delachaux & Niestlé, Neuchâtel (in German: Der Aufbau der Wirklichkeit beim Kinde. Klett, Stuttgart 1975).

Piaget J (1959) La naissance de l'intelligence chez l'enfant. Delachaux & Niestlé, Neuchâtel (in German: Das Erwachen der Intelligenz beim Kinde. Klett, Stuttgart 1975).

Rand ML (1996) As it was in the beginning: The significance of infant bonding in the development of self and relationships. J Child Youth Care 10:1–8.

Reich E, Zornanszky E (1997) Lebensenergie durch sanfte Bioenergetik. Kösel, München.

Reich W (1951) Armoring in a newborn infant. Orgone Energy Bull III (3):121–138.

Reich W (1933) Charakteranalyse (reprinted Kiepenheuer & Witsch, Köln 1989).

Rice R (1979) The effects of the Rice Infant Sensorimotor Stimulation Treatment on the development of high-risk infants. In Newborn Behavioral Organization: Nursing, Research and Implications. Liss, New York.

Spitz RA (1945) Hospitalism. An inquiry into the genesis of psychiatric conditions in early childhood. Psychoanal Study Child 1:53.

Spitz RA (1946) Hospitalism. A follow-up report. Psychoanal Study Child 2:113.

Spitz RA [1946) Anaclitic Depression. Psychoanal Study Child 2:313.

Spitz RA (1950) Anxiety in infancy: A study of its manifestation in its first year of life. Int J Psychoanal 31:138.

Stern D (1953) Ueber Verhaltens- und Charakterstörungen bei Kindern und Jugendlichen. Rascher, Zürich.

Stern D (1997) Mutter und Kind. Die erste Beziehung (original: The First Relationship: Infant and Mother 1977). Klett-Cotta, Stuttgart.

Verny T (1993) The Secret Life of the Unborn Child. Warner Books, London.

Velten H, Walter B (1997) Harmonische Babymassage. Ravensburger Buchverlag, Ravensburg.

Walker P (1995) Baby Massage. Piatkus Publishers, London.

Wendelstadt S (1998) Emotional first-aid – Healing a birth trauma. Bioenerget Anal 9:85–96.

Ventling, Christa D. (1930), 2 children, 3 grandchildren, studied chemistry at the University of Lausanne, Switzerland, and biochemistry at the University of Oxford, where she obtained a DPhil in 1957. After being active in medically oriented scientific research for many years she took up the study of psychology at the University of Basel, Switzerland, where she graduated in 1987. She worked in a psychiatric out-patient clinic before starting on her own as a psychotherapist. By 1995 she had completed her training as a bioenergetic therapist. Her main interest focuses on neuropsychobiology and unaltered from the time she was active in biochemical research, the origin of matter. She lives near Basel, Switzerland, where she has a private practice. She is a member of the editorial board of *Bioenergetic Analysis.*

Dr. phil. Christa D. Ventling, Holbeinstrasse 65, CH–4051 Basel (Switzerland)

Ventling CD (ed): Childhood Psychotherapy. A Bioenergetic Approach.
Basel, Karger, 2001, pp 19–22

Improving Bonding using Bioenergetics and Sensory Assessments: A Clinical Case Report

Vincentia Schroeter

'Do you have some bioenergetic technique you can use to help me feel closer to my unborn baby?' This question was asked by a long-term client who was 8 months pregnant. She was worried because she did not feel any bond to the life she carried inside her.

Pre-Natal Bonding

Bioenergetic Intervention

In response to her question I had her put one hand on her heart and one hand on her belly and breathe deeply. This bioenergetic technique deepens the breathing and increases the energetic charge, which often allows emotional feelings to surface. The two feelings that emerged were grief and fear. With the help of this exercise, it became clear that she was still grieving over the loss of her first baby, who had died after 5.5 months gestation.

Releasing one feeling that is held back often allows one to become aware of other feelings and to gain insights [Lowen, 1975]. After releasing some of her grief my client became aware of two fears. She feared becoming attached to a baby who might again die and also feared that her husband would focus all his attention on the new baby and forget about her. This second fear was interesting to me because often it is the father who feels anxiety about being excluded when a baby joins the family.

Examining her anxiety about being excluded led my client to explore how her own birth disrupted her family. After my client was born, her mother was preoccupied with other matters and her father was sad and detached. Her parents married reluctantly and were never closely connected emotionally.

As a child she felt this lack of connection between her parents, and now she feared that she and her husband would draw apart with the birth of their child. Breathing into her heart and belly first helped her to express grief and fear and then to have compassion for herself in light of her past. As her fears made more sense to her, the warmth in her heart increased and she felt more trust in her capacity to love. She had opened up the connection, literally and emotionally, between the child she was, the child she carried, and her own heart. She appeared relieved at the end of this session.

Post-Natal Bonding

Sensory Preference Intervention

My client returned to therapy when her new-born was 3 weeks old. She suffered moderate postpartum depression. Her predominant feelings were shock and distress over a painful childbirth and ambivalence and frustration toward her new role as a parent. She expressed dismay over, 'how much work a baby takes'. I was concerned because she appeared overwhelmed and detached from her baby.

According to the research of Stanley Greenspan et al. [1995], there are differences in how infants and children take in, perceive, and respond to sensations for each sensory system. Using their work as a starting point, I developed my own measures of sensory perceptions and responses. I used these measures in research to compare the visual and auditory sensory styles of mothers and their infants. I used the results of this research to design sensory style assessment tools for my clinical psychotherapy practice.

I was hoping that by using these assessment tools, my client would get to know and find more pleasure interacting with her baby. According to Greenspan's developmental-structuralist model [Greenspan, 1980], the new-born baby needs help from her caretaker to self-regulate and to take an interest in the world. Indeed, the more time that is spent in loving contact, the more the brain develops the capacity to be both calm and alert [Porges, 1997]. It is only during a calm and alert state that productive learning and satisfying interpersonal contact take place.

Session One

In order to help this mother tune in to the unique qualities of her baby, we tested the baby for preferred carrying position, sound preference and speed of rocking preference. I had the mother hold her 3-week-old baby in three positions, horizontal, at a 45-degree angle, and at a vertical or 90-degree angle. As the mother had already discovered, the baby appeared calmest and most alert in the vertical, over-the-shoulder position. I praised this new mother for her insight, which was reassuring to her. Next we tested the baby for sound preference and found that the baby liked the fastest and highest voice over the lower, slower voice. During the rocking, the baby preferred her mother to rock her with the fastest movements. At the end of this session, the mother remarked, 'I thought it was interesting that she responded to my voice so well, I didn't know she listened so much, and that she has preferences! The rocking – that she likes the faster movement, I didn't realise that.'

Session Two

Two weeks later, mother and baby came in for another session. The mother reported still feeling ambivalent about the baby. She resented feeling controlled by the baby's apparent need to eat every hour. When I held the baby over my shoulder and the baby squirmed, the mother said, 'See, she has eaten and she is being held and she is still not happy.' The mother asked if too much holding could 'spoil' a child. I told her that you cannot spoil a child in the 1st year of life and I intervened to help the mother understand what the baby was trying to communicate.

I applied what we had learned the previous session during the sensory assessment. This baby liked a high fast sound and fast rocking and movement. I got up out of the chair and danced actively around the room with the baby adding a high fast singing voice. The mother looked at the baby's face and remarked, 'she looks happy!' After all this activity the baby became calm. The mother now understood that the baby was not really hungry every hour, but squirmed because she was bored from not getting enough activity. We discussed ways that she and her husband could provide some type of active stimulation so their child would not be under-aroused. Our work helped her to realise that the baby was different from her or her husband. She remarked, 'We have an active baby with two mellow parents.'

As Karen [1998] says, 'The fundamental message of temperament research is that people are inherently different, and that those differences need to be tolerated and respected.' I would add that it is only in understanding and respecting these differences in preferences that parents and children can become securely attached, sensu Bowlby [1988].

Session Three

My client returned when her baby was 3 months old. I was relieved to see that she had gotten over her postpartum depression and was much happier as a mother. As she engaged in a long session of cooing in a high voice, her delighted baby smiled and imitated her sounds. Both mother and baby brightened and it was lovely to watch them go back and forth, interacting with such mutual pleasure. When a baby is about 3 months old, parents often experience a 'falling in love' with their infant, which I was delighted to witness in my client. As the mother recovered physically and hormonally from childbirth, and was supported in her task to become a loving mother, she appeared calmer and happier. At the end of this session she looked warmly at her baby and gushed, 'I love her and she is so much joy.'

Discussion

A combination of bioenergetic and sensory assessment techniques was used to help a concerned new mother establish a bond with her baby. The bioenergetic technique utilised deep breathing to help connect her heart to the unborn child in her belly. Although she initially experienced an ambivalent attachment due to postpartum depression and lack of experience, sensory preference interventions helped her to understand her new-born baby and to improve their relationship. By the time the baby was 3 months old, this mother had found her own way toward establishing a secure attachment with her baby.

References

Bowlby R (1988) A Secure Base: Parent-Child Attachment and Healthy Human Development. Basic Books, New York.

Greenspan SI (1980) The Development of the Ego: Implications for personality theory, psychopathology, and the psychotherapeutic process. International University Press, Madison.

Greenspan SI (1995) The Challenging Child. Addison-Wesley, Reading.

Karen R (1998) Becoming Attached. Oxford University Press, Oxford.

Lowen A (1975) Bioenergetics. Simon & Schuster, New York.

Porges SW (1997) Emotion: An evolutionary by-product of the neural regulation of the autonomic nervous system; in Carter CS, Lederhendler II (eds): The Integrative Neurobiology of Affiliation. New York Academy of Sciences, New York, pp 62–77.

Schroeter, Vincentia (1950), married, 1 child, holds a BA from San Francisco State University (1973), an MA from the University of San Francisco (1975) and is currently a PhD candidate at Summit University. She completed her training as a bioenergetic therapist in 1980. Besides seeing private patients in her practice she also teaches bioenergetics to trainees at the San Diego Institute for Bioenergetic Analysis. She consults on addictions. Her special psychotherapeutic interests involve integrating bioenergetics with early attachment issues and blending bioenergetics with self-psychology. On these topics she has published several articles since 1994 in the *Black Butte* Journal. She says she loves sports, dancing and teaching and most of all her family. She is a member of the editorial board of *Bioenergetic Analysis.*

Vincentia Schroeter, 1407 Stratford Court No. 2, Del Mar, CA 92014 (USA)

Ventling CD (ed): Childhood Psychotherapy. A Bioenergetic Approach.
Basel, Karger, 2001, pp 23–31

Bioenergetic Duos – Uncovering Deficits in Mother-Child Relationships

Jens Kühntopp[1], *Vita Heinrich*

Introduction

In these times characterised by a great deal of social and economical insecurity we see more and more mothers feeling helpless or confused about caring for their children. The reasons are many: some women may be too young, too immature when becoming mothers, too preoccupied with their economic survival, living in problematic relationships, or they may present other deficiencies. Many of them lack models to teach them natural bodily attitudes and gestures, what is right or wrong concerning emotional and physical contact with their child, his rhythms of eating, sleeping and 'socialising'. We know that early disturbances are based on low or non-existing sensitivity and responsiveness in primary relationships (parent-child interaction). Eventually the parent, mostly the mother, seeks help; more often than not it is the child's eccentric behaviour at home or at school which sets the scene and requires a medical and/or psychological examination followed with whatever treatment needs arise.

Children grow to responsible adults by passing through well-characterised stages. Lowen [1975] emphasises the fundamental *needs* of each stage which must be fulfiled and spells them out as *The Rights of the Child*. Thus, the child from birth on has a right to exist and to be taken care of correspondingly. He has a right to be nourished physically and emotionally, to be supported in his needs to become autonomous and independent, to experience his limitations, to return to and use the nearness of the mother whenever necessary,

[1] The work described here is part of the requirement for graduation in psychology from the University of Osnabrück, Germany.

the right to have desires and wishes, to express his will, to have an opinion of his own, to find his sexuality through identification with the parent of the same sex and the allowance to love the parent of the opposite sex. The starting basis for all this is the attachment to his mother [Bowlby, 1969] in the very beginning from where he can venture out as he develops.

With emotionally disturbed children the fundamental rights of a human being are often found to have been neglected or curtailed in the early years of life. Bowlby [1969] states that a similarity between the inner processes and the behaviour of an individual can be discovered so that the recording of the behaviour works as a guide for the parallel mental processes. The behaviour of the child is always in response to his caretaker, which usually is the mother. To assess the quality of the interaction of the child with his mother or with his surroundings seems to us of utmost priority in order to start adequate treatment.

Main stream methods of psychotherapy use mostly questionnaires to assess the degree and quality of the disturbance and use *verbal* interventions for the therapy proper. These take on the form of individual psychotherapy for the mother and the child or family therapy for parents and children together. Such psychotherapy methods may be time-consuming and therefore not very economical. Also, they leave out an important aspect, e.g. the *emotional* and *physical* contact between mother and child. In our opinion it is precisely the careful and detailed observation of the *interactional* quality of mother and child over a certain time period which is needed for a correct diagnosis of the deficits. Only after analysing the observations can we devise means to treat. It requires a perceptive psychotherapist trained in bodily expression having a solid background experience in child development. A further important prerequisite, however, is the proper diagnostic tool.

A body-oriented assessment and treatment method involving both mother and child and allowing a fair diagnosis of the problems, so far has not been described. It occurred to us that some bioenergetic exercises, although originally designed for adults, could be adapted to specific situations. Halsen [1992] did that in his psychiatric clinic in Fredrikstad, Norway. He designed and successfully tried out specific bioenergetic exercises for severely traumatised or otherwise deficient young children. He emphasised that working with disturbed children is a bodily affair. The child's bodily reactions are the message the therapist must understand and respond to. Thus, he established a warm, supportive atmosphere, offered structure and containment where there was none, promoted attachment and growth. The basis for this was the establishment of a relationship between the needy child with a caring adult, the milieu therapist. Halsen's concept was to use well-defined bioenergetic exercises which, on a physical and emotional level, could give the child what he had been lacking earlier.

Since the child is dependent on his mother for survival, it is only logical that one should have a look at both of them in interaction. Since bioenergetic exercises could be adapted to children as Halsen [1992] had done, we felt we could adapt them to 'partners', here to the mother-child duo. The child experiences himself as a physical unity with boundaries and the mother as a separate being with its own physical boundaries. On these boundaries contact and interaction take place allowing such experiences as independence, freedom or nearness. Problems in this relationship become obvious and deficits can be spelled out. The insights gained are the basis for a change to a better relationship.

Taking into account the developmental steps of children and the respective needs of each period, we selected a series of exercises from Halsen [1992] which we modified into interaction exercises for mother and child. When these exercises are presented to a mother-child duo, the observation and analysis of how each one of them reacted can provide clues to the quality of their interaction and the deficits of this interaction. In the following, we describe the exercises and our way of proceeding.

Bioenergetic Exercises for Mother and Child

Grounding Exercises

Any grounding exercises in different positions (upright, using a support like leaning against a wall, or lying down) can be used and varied. Grounding by walking: mother and child are asked to walk on their toes/heels, on the outside/inside of the foot or fast/slow, for example. Walking exercises sensitize the body. These exercises are therefore placed at the beginning of a session. Exercises with mother and child leaning upright against a wall or lying on the back, give the feeling of support and security, especially in the back. To do the exercises without fear and with a feeling of security is important. The observer must be prepared to perceive any arising emotions.

Co-Ordination

Bicycle riding: Mother and child are lying on their backs, legs up in the air with the soles of their feet pressing against each other. They begin to move their legs in a circle-like motion. Both mother and child can decide how fast or how slow they want to go and move together. Both are careful not to lose contact. A similar exercise can be done with the hands: Mother and child are sitting on the floor, pressing the palms of their hands together. Now both begin to move their arms in a circle-like fashion, slowly or wildly as they wish. In this exercise mother and child become aware of how they move their bodies together. The rhythm of their movements reflects the quality of their interaction.

Feeling Strength

Here the child can try out his strength. He decides himself how strong he wants to be, and for how long and when to give in. The child is lying on his back and is asked to resist the mother's effort to turn him around. Having shown his strength, he may give in to the mother and roll over. The same principle can be used, while the child is on his knees on the floor with this hands firmly planted in front of him and resisting his mother to push him over. Mother and child can also change places, so that the child tries to push the mother over. This exercise shows how the mother uses her power, whether and how she accepts the child's decisions. If she uses her power in a self-centred way, not giving the child a chance, not respecting his needs, overstepping the limits of her child, he will react. The reaction can be aggressive or submissive. Thus, it also shows how the child perceives his strength.

Confidence Exercises

The child lies down on his back and makes himself stiff, while the mother lifts him up to a standing position. The exercise can be reversed, so that both start from the standing position. The mother is feeling the full weight of the child in her arms. She is carrying the responsibility, while the child is trusting her arms. A variation to this is for the mother to guide the child with closed eyes around the room. This exercise can be reversed, so that the child guides the mother; here attention must be paid that the child does this in control of himself. For it is a lot of fun to let the mother run against a wall or against another person. A further variation to the theme of trust is this exercise: while the child is lying on his back, the mother holds the child's head in her hands and moves it about very slowly and very gently. It is important to do these exercises with concentration and great caution. The quality of the interaction is expressed by the observed trusting of the child in his mother and also by the degree of sensitivity and cautiousness.

Qualities of Touching

The mother touches the child, e.g. during a massage. Afterwards, the child describes his sensations. Then the child touches the mother, who also reports her sensations. The awareness of the body, the sensation and the verbal expression of emotions and sensations are trained with these exercises. They help mother and child to be aware of, give words to, and try out different kinds of touch.

Nurturing Exercises

These are not exercises in the true sense, but rather protecting, nurturing and loving motions of the mother towards the child. Thus, the mother may cover the child with a blanket and give him a very gentle massage for example. It increases the child's ability to be receptive and feel pleasure. The nurturing behaviour of the mother shows, if and how much she is willing to give.

The Setting

Of course, the setting we describe in the following could be adapted to individual needs. One can work with one dyad only or with two. If more than one dyad is in a session at a time, this allows the additional analysis of the children, or the mothers towards each other, e.g. the effect of each dyad onto the other. In our report here we describe our work with two dyads at the same time.

The exercises were done in a gym room. It contained mats and blankets and had three video cameras installed. Each session was recorded on videotape. (Since our goal was also to evaluate in a scientific way the interactional exercises and their effectiveness regarding the quality of the mother-child relationship, the sessions recorded on videotape were later analysed. Thus, of each dyad six videotapes were made, each analysed by two independent raters, using two especially constructed questionnaires, one for the mother and one for the child. Results were factor-analysed and the inter-rater reliability was calculated [Lienert and Raatz, 1994]. The results will be published elsewhere.) The therapist led the exercises for the two dyads simultaneously. The duration of the session of approximately 1 h was adapted to the child's ability to concentrate on the session. The intensity of the session was carefully monitored. Exercises were proposed in a joyful way, like playing games, so that the children were free to take part without pressure. We always remembered our aim, which is to bring mother and child into a joyful, individual and 'natural' relationship. The order of the exercises was pre-determined: we began with grounding and continued in the following order with exercises on co-ordination, feeling strength, confidence, qualities of touching and ending with nurturing. The exercises were decreasing in physical activity and ending with quiet time, which corresponds to a reversed order of the stages of child development. At the end of each session the therapist wrote a short protocol for each dyad, registering the exercises and his observations. Six sessions were held altogether in weekly intervals.

The Dyads

Dyad 1: Albert with His Mother Angela

Albert was brought to our psychiatric clinic at the age of 7 years and 7 months. He was diagnosed according to ICD-10 to have the symptoms of F 92 (combined social and affective behaviour disorder) and F 90.1 (attention deficit hyperactivity disorder). He received no medication. Albert was apparently extremely restless and agitated; in school, he did not respect rules or laws, and in order to get what he wanted he would scream, behave wildly and beat around and he had no motivation to learn. With his behaviour he disturbed both class and teacher and gradually became completely intolerable. Albert was an only child. His parents, Angela and Adam, were both working full-time. The maternal grandparents were taking care of Albert during the week. They felt that they had to make up for the lack of time the parents spent with the child and so they gave Albert a lot of attention, granting him every wish, not setting any borders. Angela complained about the behaviour of her parents and also felt that they allowed Albert the things that she and her husband would not allow him. Her husband, Adam, was a mechanical construction worker whose job forced him to be away almost the entire week. On weekends he was available for his son. Since the bioenergetic exercise sessions took place during the week, due to his work obligation, he was excluded from participating in the sessions, which he regretted. So the mother agreed to come to the dyad sessions.

Within the first sessions it became obvious that Angela had great difficulties in setting limits to Albert. He, on the other hand, blatantly sought the confrontation with others, provoking his mother and disturbing the other dyad. We had the impression he was continuously trying to attract attention and to find a trustworthy base for security. Angela's repertoire in behavioural responses towards Albert was found to be rather limited. She tried in vain to give nearness and security – with a few exceptions, Albert would refuse her attempts. In the fourth session, Albert was so obstructive in his behaviour that the therapist had to interfere as the mother could not cope anymore with her son. At the sixth session, Albert expressed his regrets that the sessions had come to an end. This came as a surprise because in the past sessions it was never obvious that Albert enjoyed what he was asked to do. On the contrary, it seemed more and more like a duty he had to fulfil. We concluded therefore that for a child like Albert six sessions are not enough. Regrettably, we could not continue the sessions for various reasons.

Dyad 2: Betty with Her Mother Barbara

Betty was admitted to our clinic as an in-patient at the age of 8 years and 3 months. Her diagnosis according to the ICD-10 was F 92 (combined social and affective behaviour disorder) and F 90.0 (simple activity and attention deficits). No medication was prescribed. In school and at home, Betty was disturbing whatever activity was going on. She was lying very often, did not pay attention to what was being said, her homework was not done properly which increased the tension between her and her mother Barbara to the point where Barbara became desperate. Betty was a middle child, she had an older sister and a younger brother. Her father Bernie was addicted to alcohol and gambling and took no responsibility in his family. He was mostly absent. Betty did not have a good relationship with her father.

During the first session Betty and Barbara were both rather restless and excited due to the newness of it all, but in all further sessions they calmed down. Compared to the rather unruly Albert and Angela dyad they formed a quiet counterpart. Barbara was cool, withdrawn and uninviting towards Betty. She found it very difficult to touch her child, to feel her body. Betty, on the other hand, appreciated and loved the physical contact with her mother, which increased in intensity with every session. At the beginning of the third session Barbara verbalised her feelings which a certain exercise in the previous session had set free. It was an exercise where Barbara had to cradle Betty's head gently in her hands. She said: 'It was so terrible, I went home and just wanted to die, I did not care for anything anymore.' This experience shook up Barbara. After that she and Betty enjoyed the exercises more and more. The physical contact and the entire relationship between the two became more intensive and harmonious. Shortly after the termination of the sessions, Betty was able to leave the clinic. Her mother Barbara decided to go into therapy.

Discussion and Conclusions

Disturbances in the early interaction between mother and child are thought to be the cause for later neurotic and psychotic disorders. Reich [1983] emphasised the importance of a good mother-child interaction from birth on in order to prevent 'armouring' as he called it, which in his thinking set the stage for later neuroses and psychoses, but he never spelled out how he understood prevention of armouring. To hope that there exists a method to eliminate future psychopathological problems would lead into never-ending arguing and has little basis with reality. More likely we should encourage therapists and researchers to try out various forms. The child, after all, comes into this world equipped with his own genetic make-up, the mother has her own and the two of them must now 'dance' together [Stern, 1985] and all this under the influence of the surrounding emotional and social environment. Early communication is non-verbal, it is based on empathy, appreciation, acceptance, friendliness, warm-hearted feelings, reciprocal exchange and mirroring of feelings between mother and child. The mother responds in an appropriate manner to the body signals of the child. If she does not or cannot 'read' the child, his needs are frustrated, he becomes angry, sad, desperate and in the end gives up in resignation. Since aggressiveness or resignation in a later stage of development is often a reason for sending a child to a psychiatric institution, we became interested in diagnosing the problems as early as possible. Early diagnosis with subsequent treatment may help to diminish the severity of a later adult form of disturbance or even prevent it. For the moment being this remains hypothetical, although our elaboration of two short case histories here seems promising. Long-term studies would definitely be needed to validate this hypothesis.

Our investigation is a diagnostic procedure providing extensive information about the mother, the child and their interactions. From observing bodily interactions we can deduct assumptions about the psychic, social and emotional state. Such information was collected in vivo, i.e. live and directly, and furthermore, in very few sessions. The procedure is effective, economical and a worthy addition to the classical diagnostics of intelligence, perception, personality and family organisation. We would be most pleased if our work would find many imitators.

References

Bowlby J (1969) Attachment and Loss, vol 1: Attachment. Basic Books, New York.

Halsen AW (1992) Bioenergetic work with children: Experiences in a child psychiatric unit. J Int Inst Bioenerget Anal 5:30–44.

Lienert GA, Raatz U (1994) Testaufbau und Testanalyse, 5. Auflage. Psychologische Verlagsunion; Weinheim.

Lowen A (1975) Bioenergetics. Simon & Schuster, New York (in German: Bioenergetik. Therapie der Seele durch Arbeit mit dem Körper. Rowohlt, Reinbek, 1988).

Reich W (1983) Children of the Future. On the Prevention of Sexual Pathology. Farrar, Straus, Giroux; New York.

Stern D (1985) The Interpersonal World of the Infant. Basic Books, New York.

Kühntopp, Jens (1968), married, 4 children, graduated at the University of Osnabrück in 1997 as a clinical psychologist. He works with children and adolescents, using mainly concepts of the systemic family approach, together with bioenergetic elements. His experience covers work with children of divorced parents, children with attention deficit disorders and phobias.

Jens Kühntopp, Auf der Heide 8, D–32257 Bünde (Germany)

Heinrich, Vita (1955), mother of 1 child, holds a doctorate in psychology from the University of Osnabrück, Germany. She has been working in a private practice since more than 10 years. She completed her training as a bioenergetic therapist in 1991. She teaches diagnostics and bioenergetic analysis at the University of Osnabrück where she is also engaged in research. She has published a book and several articles on various subjects and is one of the co-editors of *Bioenergetic Analysis.*

Dr. phil. Vita Heinrich, Humboldtstrasse 14a, D–49047 Osnabrück (Germany)

Ventling CD (ed): Childhood Psychotherapy. A Bioenergetic Approach.
Basel, Karger, 2001, pp 32–40

The Blue Ball Intervention: Integrating Bioenergetics into a Children's Acute Care Psychiatric Unit

Tom Wills

Introduction

Descriptive material on the implementation of bioenergetic approaches in psychotherapy with younger children is hard to find. Arnt Halsen in 'The Journal' (of the International Institute for Bioenergetic Analysis; reprinted in this book) laid down a cornerstone when describing his work with children in an in-patient setting. Extending Halsen's work, this article describes my own application of bioenergetic concepts in interventions with children out of control. The setting in this writing is a 16-bed in-patient acute care children's unit (part of a small private psychiatric hospital).

The majority of the children in our unit are boys (average male/female ratio is 10/1, age 5–11 years), having suffered major nurturing deprivations in their first few years. We find a high percentage of drug abuse by their mothers during pregnancy. In addition, almost every patient has had a physical or sexual trauma. Thus we see the standard DSM IV Axis One Diagnoses with a high percentage of aggressive oppositional defiant conduct disorder in the older children. The children's stay in the unit averages 23 days, ranging from 4 days to 6 months. Medical treatment in the unit centres primarily on pharmaceutical strategies managed by the child psychiatrist. As Programme Director, I am in charge of the infrastructure for the behaviour programme that supplements the medical modalities and provides practical strategies for the children to utilise upon leaving the hospital for home or another placement.

The Behavioural Programme

The programme is structured on a behavioural model; each child receives up to five points per activity. Activities are highly structured and are both cognitive and emotive in nature. Group work is designed to provide practice in interaction, role-play, and playful, creative insight into their social dynamics. Packets of assignments are prepared that utilise materials familiar to children in school. Homework is also provided to add an appropriate discipline to the child's routine. A child can earn up to 100 points per day with rewards and certificates given out each evening. The point system is strengthened three times a day through 'point talks' during which the children's progress is reviewed. Children are not given negative points. The specific rationale for each point is described to the children. For example, a child is told that he attained three points for lunch and the reason why. A detailed warning/time-out system is a major intervention strategy of the point system. This warning system is spelled out in a set of explicit guidelines known to staff and patients. The system starts with 1-min time-outs for minor disruptive behaviour. The time-out is often accomplished by having the child sit separately and quietly in the room in which the particular activity is taking place. Time-out may increase up to 5 min, and at this point the child is removed from the activity. There are generally two warnings before a time-out begins. When the child is unable to self-control with the time-outs, the child is brought to the 'Quiet Room' (see below) for an extended period; if the child is assessed as able to proceed with the activity, the necessary material is brought to him/her.

In the following I describe the development and implementation of particular bioenergetic interventions in conjunction with the therapeutic behavioural/pharmaceutical programme of controlling the children's tensions and aggressiveness.

Integrating Bioenergetic Interventions

Setting the Stage

Early in the development of the children's unit programme it became clear that music/dance and movement sessions were very helpful in releasing the tension that these children struggled with. According to the current bioenergetic theory, tensions are due to blocked emotions located in distinct parts of the body, which can be released by the use of specific bioenergetic exercises or body interventions. Thus the plan was to combine play therapy with bioenergetic techniques to find a way to contribute productively to the child's ability to self-regulate. For this purpose, first the Quiet Room was redesigned into a friendly space. One wall was padded with two-inch foam and covered with bright blue material. The rest of the room was trimmed in a soothing green; a large decorative border of whales and dolphins was placed near the ceiling. For hygienic reasons the floor was left covered with linoleum. Acoustical tile was added to the ceiling the 2nd year to deaden sound. Second, it became clear that certain guidelines were needed in order to make sure that the bioenergetic activities in the Quiet Room followed a standard procedure maintained across shifts of staff. Thus I developed a policy and procedure document known as *Emotional Management Intervention* (EMI). The EMI policy was reviewed by the treatment team consisting of the director/child psychiatrist, nurse manager and myself. The collaborative process, clear rationale plus a step by step structure were needed to make the intervention safe for all parties. The EMI among others contains these important guidelines.

(1) There is an understanding that this intervention is not a behaviour model, and that it is not a reward for 'good' behaviour or for taking the medication, for example.

(2) The vision of EMI is clarified as a one-time 5-min intervention to be followed by a quiet time in the Quiet Room. This gives the staff time to evaluate the success of the intervention. If the child is unable to self-regulate and follow basic directions; a nurse is called to evaluate the need for medication or other strategies.

(3) The staff must be aware of the limitations of the child and know the specific child-centred treatment goals developed by the treatment team.

(4) There is a staff educational component to the intervention. This consists of an educational packet with six hands-on training sessions and an observation check-off sheet. The completion of this training qualifies the staff to deal with children independently without the consultation of the nurse in charge.

(5) Sessions may include two staff members per child.

(6) Sessions are interventions, to be used when a child needs to regain the ability to self-regulate and thus rejoin peers in the programme.

Specific Bioenergetic Exercises

At first I explored simple basic grounding exercises with the children removed to the Quiet Room. Grounding allowed the children to move out of their mental confusion. These interventions received positive reactions from the patient and the staff, in particular from the psychiatrist. Having thus gained the confidence of the professional staff, I was very often called in to 'help get this kid together'. Training of staff members who have had no experience of their own with bioenergetics was more problematic. I tried to overcome their doubts by introducing a large, very light and soft 24-inch 'blue ball', a very familiar object. The ball was simply thrown back and forth in a variety of patterns. This helped staff members to interact more willingly with the agitated patients. Sometimes a small range of exercises was added to the intervention. The exercises were kept quite simple and very safe. The ball became a distracting and calming mechanism to the child's behaviour, as it required perceptual focus connected to physical movement. Thus, the use of the blue ball provided a whole-body exercise which transformed the chaotic behaviour of the out-of-control child into an organised game.

We worked basically with the following group of exercises.

Grounding Exercise

Almost all the interventions are done in stocking feet. We have instigated a rule: if you want to kick the ball you have to be in stocking feet. (With extremely agitated patients who cannot make contact and are safe enough, this rule is given some latitude.) One of the favourite grounding exercises is to bounce the ball and hop from right to left, or to count to ten on each foot. This gives an added bit of self-confidence. Holding the ball in both hands and balancing on one foot, then challenging the child to bend the knee creates an ideal 'win-win' grounding game. We try to follow the rule that for most children brought into the Quiet Room 'less is best' work.

Releasing Exercises

For the most part these children are angry and frightened and release and discharge of their tensions occurs naturally. The critical point is to make contact with them, so that they can lower the tension and begin reorganising by establishing a safe relationship with an adult. The children's intense energy puts significant demands on the staff members' own ability to tolerate lots of energy for short periods of time, while remaining in contact with their ego/feelings. This is why the EMI has remained a short, specific, goal-oriented task. In these children almost all the energy is in the upper part of the body and they are often releasing it by yelling or swearing. The best place to begin is, therefore, right here, though often the timing is a very delicate moment and inflections need to match with respect and dignity. Throwing the ball or kicking it are the two exercises that have been the most successful. Both these interventions demonstrate that children will naturally discharge through their feet while activating the aggressive areas in the upper and lower back. Depending on the individual patient, the ball is directed at the wall or the staff. This is a judgement call with different outcomes. Because the EMI is used to organise the child and not increase the child's chaotic state, the inanimate character of the wall is most often used.

The key here is not only to help the child feel safe and understand that we can tolerate his or her primitive tensions and out-of-control behaviour, but help the child understand that this state is not effective in the long term and that there are other ways to release this energy. Therefore, following the active releasing exercise, a 5-min verbal and supportive intervention was found to be a good way to do our educational instruction, keeping in mind that it must be at the child's level of understanding. This time is as important as the active intervention. It is the time when the child may be able to accept some holding and soothing by the staff as delineated by Winnicott [1958]. This concept of the child's ability to accept holding and soothing is crucial to overcoming the developmental shortcomings of these children. The staff member must remain in contact with the child and not re-stimulate but rather support the child. Here, even the economy of words is significant in that language has significant energy and contact. Often the simplest of statements is more than adequate, such as 'Geeeee...you were mad.... At the end you were having a good time...'

Progressive Exercises

I found that helping children reach their full developmental stage is the most difficult area to educate the staff about. Often a child in the Quiet Room demonstrates less than his age behaviour. We see regression and also complex dissociation [Herman, 1992]. Dissociative states are often fleeting, can be frightening, misunderstood or not even noticed by the staff. Loss of contact with the patient occurs as the result of a mixture of judgement, fear, and need to control on the part of the staff. However, the regressed patient is honoured as well as dissociative states are given time to come to an increased healthy contact state. Time to explore is important while the staff makes contact at the highest ego functioning. Because so many of our patients had major trauma in their history, we found – as Halsen [1992] – a great need to regress. Progressive exercises are geared to assist the child to his correct developmental age. Therefore, when children fall down in a regressed state or end up on the mat, foot contact is one of the must successful exercises, once it is clear that the child feels safe. This activity starts with the child's own feet on the padded wall, then may progress to the child's feet making contact with the staff's feet in a playful contact activity.

Clinical Examples

Prior to implementing EMI, the front-line staff, called mental health associates (MHAs), typically have made at least one time-out intervention or, with the nurse, an additional assessment, and agreed the patient would benefit from an EMI. This procedure has an added benefit in that the EMI gives the MHA a greater role and increased positive contact with the child. In the descriptions of the interventions that follow, the implementation is described in the context of the child's particular diagnosis and behaviours. In the first two examples, I employ the basic EMI procedure, in the second instance the EMI is combined with some additional reframing interactions, e.g. techniques that help the child perceive reality in a new and more productive way. The third example demonstrates the use of the EMI as part of the comprehensive treatment plan. All names are fictitious and historical information has been modified to protect the identity of the patients.

Albert is 9 years old. This is his third hospitalisation. He lives with his biological mother and three siblings; his father has re-entered the family just recently. Before this admission he became obsessed by his aunt's baby trying to attack her and the baby at one point with a knife. He remained with us for 3 months and was discharged to home with day treatment and additional services in place. His DSM-IV diagnosis upon discharge was attention deficit hyperactivity disorder (ADHD), combined type, 314.01, disruptive behaviour disorder not otherwise specified (NOS), 312.9, opposition defiant, schizoid, affect-depressive type. Albert has been angry, defiant and intrusive throughout the morning school programme. He has been placed in the Quiet Room and is yelling foul language, banging on the wall. He did not want to be in the room and has refused to take medication. I had worked with Albert many times in a variety of activity settings. When I entered the Quiet Room, the very first thing he yells is 'I don't want that ...blue ball.' I say nothing and go over to the locked door and remove the ball and start bouncing it back and forth with the MHA. This has become a near standard first move and seems to create a calming effect, spreading out the negative transference from me towards the MHA, while clearly being an enticing redirecting object. At one point the ball is bounced to Albert who angrily throws it to me; we now have him engaged, and he continues the ball throwing until the feeling of play emerges. At this point the rules of the EMI are lightly reviewed with the child. One of the key guidelines is that if the child is unable to sit quietly after the intervention, then he may have to take medication. The EMI procedure states that if there is any question about taking medications, a nurse is to make the final judgement as well as to when the patient is to return to the programme.

Tonya, 10 years old, is a depressed, angry girl who impulsively strikes out and becomes aggressive when she does not get her way. This is her first hospitalisation. She was living in a foster home after becoming unmanageable. There was anecdotal information that she was abused and had witnessed the suicide of her biological father as a young child. Her stay with us was an uncommonly long time of 9 months, complicated by her legal as well as clinical picture. She was discharged to a long-term residential treatment setting. Her diagnosis upon discharge was ADHD, adjustment disorder with mixed disturbance of emotion and conduct, 309.4, and post-traumatic stress disorder, 309.81. Midway through her stay with us, Tonya, when she is held accountable, often falls to the floor and 'temper tantrums' follow for long periods of time. She is in the Quiet Room on the mat, pouting, refusing any directions or positive contact. Plenty of space is allowed and after a while a staff member and I roll the ball back and forth between us. Slowly Tonya joins in and starts to make babyish sounds and is soothing herself, making small contact with each of us. At times she makes playful angry sounds at us with the ball. The energy continues to move and we talk in supportive positive statements about how good she is and how smart for example. After a short time, I state 'I wonder if Tonya is big enough to bounce the ball.' With the added energy and a few playful, more subtle directions she is on her feet and we are watching a 10-year-old girl enjoy herself in play. Almost out of the blue Tonya states, 'I want to go back to school.' At this point the rule is stated 'matter-of-factly': There is to be some quiet time on the mat; she sits down. We review with Tonya what she learned or saw during this intervention, review the scene that brought her in to the Quiet Room, and reframe her actions in a positive way. For this purpose, I have used some classic question from Psychodrama practice, 'What did you learn?...What did you see?' [Goldman, 1984] and may actually do some reframing by having the child role-play the scene that brought her into the Quiet Room. Most of the MHAs would not be able to take the intervention to this next level of insight. However, even the use of the ball itself according to the structured guidelines provides an intervention technique that may prevent the need for more intensive strategies.

Rich, an 11-year-old child, had been with us 4 months, considerably beyond our average 23-day stay. He had been in the foster care system since he was 3 years old. His foster family of 7 years recently rejected him, returning him to the Welfare Department and refused any contact with him. This is his first hospitalisation. His discharge diagnosis was ADHD, combined type 314.01, disruptive behaviour disorder NOS 312.9. Because his lack of impulse control was dangerous to others, he was placed on 'one-to-one' (e.g. a staff member is with him at all times) for many weeks. In this case we implemented the blue ball intervention three times a day and increased the intervention time to 10 min. This highly structured active period gave the patient and the staff a break from the routine and helped lower the tense impulses. In this case, some additional exercises were also utilised, but the goal here was to be as aerobic as possible and to employ a positive game or a playful style.

For Albert, Tonya and Rich, the bioenergetic intervention became a tool for re-connecting the children to their own ability to control their behaviour.

Through simple, physical and interactive techniques, more radical interventions were avoided. In addition, the children were able to relax their tensions sufficiently to contain and structure their emotions and to state goals and wishes. In bioenergetic terms [Lowen, 1975], they have reorganised themselves with the help of others, in doing so they have grounded the tensions of the body and in that process regained their self-expression.

Discussion

The introduction of bioenergetic techniques into a more cognitive and behaviourally oriented clinical setting clearly created anxiety among the staff. It was a process to implement this type of approach in a traditional hospital setting. I would argue that these two systems do not have to conflict. Rather, this study suggests that by building trust of professional staff, following a collaborative process, providing for the gentle education of support personnel, and making careful choices of non-threatening strategies, the tension between the models can be overcome and bioenergetic techniques can be successfully integrated into the clinical setting. Persuading the staff of the efficacy of the intervention and ensuring its safety required patience and understanding of their concerns. It was particularly difficult to explain the difference between bioenergetic work and other exercise interventions. However, I learned that demonstrating and explaining are best accomplished through heartfelt practical examples [Lowen, pers. commun.]. When I realised the impact that this work was having and the demands that it placed on the staff, the EMI was developed. The written guidelines provided increased credibility to the process. In turn, the policy gave structure to a staff that changed from shift to shift. While the basic intervention process has been implemented, some of the more subtle concepts are more difficult to teach in a training model. Perhaps some of the most difficult concepts to introduce into a highly behavioural model are the concepts of play and those of 'good enough' [Winnicott, 1971], because neither of these concepts is based on a reward system. In order to continue to strengthen the EMI process and to refine the potential of bioenergetic approaches, additional on-going in-service training will be needed.

Conclusion

The future for bioenergetics as part of an acute psychiatric hospital looks very promising. Its limitation is the understanding and education of the staff. Developing a policy is a significant first step in implementing any type of body-oriented intervention. Such a programme is shaped by the personal work of the trainer and the staff within such a policy. The report presented here bears witness to this.

References

Goldman E (1984) Psychodrama: Experience and Process. Kendall/Hunt, Dubuque.

Halsen A (1992) Bioenergetic work with children: Experiences in a child psychiatric unit. J Int Inst Bioenerget Anal 5:30–44.

Herman J (1992) Trauma and Recovery. Basic Books, New York.

Lowen A (1975) Bioenergetics. Penguin Books, London.

Winnicott DW (1958) Collected Papers. Tavistock, London.

Winnicott DW (1971) Playing and Reality. Basic Books, New York.

Wills, Tom (1937), married, 3 children, 1 grandchild. After obtaining his nursing degrees (RN, MSW), he started a private practice for children and adults while continuing his formation in client-centred therapy (Rogers) and in psychodrama (Moreno). He is currently in training to become a bioenergetic therapist. As a child psychotherapist he tries to combine his previously acquired behavioural experience with bioenergetic concepts. He is Programme Director for the Acute Care Children's Unit at Stony Lodge Hospital, Ossining, N.Y., USA, since 1995, where he also teaches theoretical and practical aspects of child development and play therapy in combination with bioenergetic interventions. On the side he also maintains a private practice.

Tom Wills, 21 Quaker Ridge Road, Ossining, NY 10562 (USA)

Ventling CD (ed): Childhood Psychotherapy. A Bioenergetic Approach.
Basel, Karger, 2001, pp 41–52

Bioenergetic Work with Children: Experiences from a Child Psychiatric Unit

Arnt V. Halsen

Introduction

Considering how much emphasis bioenergetics places on the influence of infancy and childhood for later character formation [Helfaer, 1988–1989 Lewis, 1976], it is astonishing how little is written about bioenergetic therapy with children. I assume that this reflects a lack of tradition and experience of working directly with youngsters in bioenergetic analysis. Wilhelm Reich himself was very occupied with infants and children, but mostly from a preventive point of view. He hoped that through changes in child upbringing and educational systems there would be less armouring and pathology in adults. With his own son Peter, he employed a kind of 'play therapy' in which he dealt directly with emotional expression and the flow of energy through contact, body games and muscle movement [Sharaf, 1983].

Reich lived and worked in Norway from 1934 to 1939, where one of his students was Dr. Nic Waal, a pioneer in Norwegian child psychiatry [Waal, 1958]. Nic Waal's Institute in Oslo is the country's most important centre for training of child psychotherapists and child psychiatric team workers. Bodily aspects of diagnosis and therapy are therefore integrated in much psychiatric work with children in Norway.

After my training at the Nic Waal Institute in 1968–1971, I became director of the child psychiatric clinic in Fredrikstad, 60 miles south of Oslo. We have a small in-patient unit for 7 children (age 7–12 years) and a kindergarten for day-treatment of 5 pre-school children. Our out-patient unit treats about 200 children and their families a year.

Residential treatment in the in-patient unit and the kindergarten is offered to severely disturbed children. In the first few years, these were psychotic/autistic or very aggressive children. We now see more borderline children and sexually and physically abused children with severe attachment problems.

To help these children one needs time. Most of the children participate in our programmes for 1–2 years, some 3 years. During this time we try to create a dependent attachment between the child and the therapist. We believe that true independence and self-reliance can be achieved only if the child has (or has had) a dependent relationship with an adult who can offer a secure base [Bowlby, 1988].

Building this kind of relationship with traumatised, rejecting, aggressive, and withdrawn children is a formidable task. Educating, supervising, and supporting the milieu therapists (psychiatric nurses and child care workers) is crucial to ensure progress. The milieu therapist's understanding of the child's dynamics, of transference issues, and of their own countertransference reactions on the one side, combined with useful therapeutic tools on the other side, seem to promote growth and healing in these wounded children.

In our clinic we establish a warm, supportive atmosphere. We offer programmes with clear structures which provide containment for our children. The structure is not based upon fixed rules but on the adult defining the limits in the relationship with the child. Responsible adults create responsible children.

Working with disturbed children is a very bodily affair. Winnicott's concepts of holding and handling are very useful in a child psychiatric unit. To promote attachment and growth this holding must go beyond stopping the acting out. In a very concrete and bodily way, we must offer warm, secure, responsible care and protection of the child and his surroundings. The milieu therapist must be able to understand and react to the emotional message in the child's bodily reactions. Bioenergetic understanding of energy concepts and the blocking and expression of emotions has been of immense value to the general development of our work [Lowen, 1975].

The Bioenergetic Program

Body therapy with our children started in 1976 with what we then called body stimulation. It was based upon physiotherapy and movement therapy (inspired by Veronica Sherborne and Rudolf Laban) and to some extent on body-oriented child psychotherapy. In the last years bioenergetic exercises designed for children have become an important part of this therapy.

We design a programme for each child with specific exercises related to the most important problems of that child. Each child has a weekly session of 15–60 min with his/her milieu therapist. The sessions take place in a room specially set up for this use with thick carpet, mattresses, and many cushions and pillows. On the wall there is a mirror which can be closed. There is no other furniture.

The programmes and the sessions are supervised by a bioenergetically trained child psychiatrist or psychologist meeting weekly with three or four milieu therapists.

The aims of the programme are both educational and therapeutic and are intertwined in the daily work with the children. Working with their deficits, filling in their lack of ordinary developmental experiences, and building up new skills are mainly educational tasks. Working with their early traumas, internalised conflicts, and suppressed feelings are more therapeutic tasks.

Above all, we need to strengthen their egos by increasing their self-awareness, self-expression, and self-possession [Lowen, 1989]. We want to create a therapeutic setting with a bioenergetic programme based on the following guiding principles:

(1) improving the children's knowledge of awareness of and contact with their bodies and their feelings;

(2) increasing their ability to express these feelings, bodily and verbally;

(3) increasing their conscious control of their emotional expressions, improving their ability to tolerate and contain emotions and tensions; helping them to see the meaning of and the reason for their emotions and reactions;

(4) building and securing their borders, physically and psychologically;

(5) reducing their tendency to split, recognising that other people are not completely bad or completely good,

(6) strengthening their identity and their ability to stand on their own feet;

(7) working with concentration and with setting and pursuing goals; developing coping mechanisms, and

(8) offering a secure base for further development of interpersonal relationships.

Categories of Bioenergetic Exercises for Children

Some of the bioenergetic exercises we use are the same we use for adults. Many exercises are modified, and some – often the more playful ones – are designed especially for children. The exercises we use have various functions in the work with a given child. I have listed twelve categories showing different functional aims for the exercises. Of course, any exercise might be used for different aims at different times.

Recognising the Body and the Body Parts

The child or the therapist points at or touches different body parts and puts names on them. It is astonishing how unaware of their bodies some of these disturbed children are even if their level of general information might be high.

Qualities of Touching

These exercises help the children to be aware of, put words to, and try out different kinds of touch (firm, soft, cold, good, and hurtful). Mostly, the therapist touches the child, who then reports his sensations and feelings. We can also let the child touch the therapist. This is often frightening to our children. They have no experience in being the active one, and they easily feel themselves as offenders. Through these exercises the children also learn to tolerate pleasure from foot massage, gentle stroking, and so on.

Feeling Bodily Strength

These exercises are developed to help the children feel they can be strong or weak, that they can hold back or give in, that they have a choice. The child is asked to lie down on his back and to resist the therapist's effort to turn him around. After he has felt his strength, he is instructed to give in to the therapist and roll over. The same principle can be used when the child is standing on hands and knees. It can be astonishing for a therapist to see and feel the great difference between the available strength in the upper part of the body and the complete lack of strength in the lower back, the pelvis, and the thigh area of sexually abused children.

The same exercises can be done by the child with the therapist lying on her back or standing on hands and knees. In this way the child is allowed to use and feel his strength in pushing an adult body.

Grounding Exercises

The whole range of known grounding exercises can be used. The therapist working with the child's feet (foot massage) can precede grounding exercises. Many of our children seem to be constantly up in the air. They are running away from themselves. Standing or lying down can be terrifying. In the standing position, the children slowly learn that their feet will support them. They also sense how to feel grounded on earth. Lying down also gives an experience of body contact with the ground. To accept the support from the ground and from the therapist at the same time makes them feel more secure. A combination of holding and grounding can be necessary [Ludwig, 1990].

Working with Borders and Boundaries

Many of these children, whether they can be classified as borderline or not, have been intruded upon by abusive, ignorant parents or other adults. The exercises in this category are very realistic. The child lays a string or a long blanket roll on the floor to mark his border and to claim his territory. The child is asked to walk around in his territory and say: 'This is mine. This belongs to me.' The child can decide if he wants to open his border, whom he wants to let in, and how long he shall stay.

Another exercise in this category involves holding the palms of the hands against the therapist's hands, sometimes to push away, sometimes to let the therapist come nearer. Often the children need to learn not to let others come too close.

Confidence Exercises

These exercises help to increase the children's trust in adults. The child is asked to lie on his back and make himself stiff while the therapist lifts him up to a standing position. The exercise can be reversed so one starts from the standing position, although this is more frightening. The therapist can also lead the child with closed eyes around the room. In another exercise, the child lies down and the therapist holds his head. The child can slowly learn to let go of control and constant watching [Lewis, 1986].

Expressive Exercises

One needs to be very careful using expressive exercises with impulsive and disorganised children. We need a very slow process so that the child can tolerate the strong feeling and gradually express them without becoming chaotic. For most of our children, it is necessary to help them identify their feelings and teach them to express their feelings. We have a chart of Donald Duck faces showing different emotional expressions: sad, angry, happy, and so forth. The child can point to the expression that corresponds to his feelings. He can try to imitate the expression and use the mirror to see his own face.

We also use playful exercises. One boy, who had a lot of suppressed anger and could speak only with a whispering voice, was able to play a barking dog. After some time, this made a dramatic difference in his voice in school and on the ward. Pillow fighting is another expressive play we use.

Control Exercises

These are designed to help the impulsive children have better control and to help the controlled children loosen up and let go. Expressing anger while maintaining control and staying in contact with the adult is a difficult and important task. To obtain this we often use very detailed prescriptions: 'Count to three', 'Hit the mattress once' or 'Look at me'.

Regressive and Progressive Exercises

Our children easily regress. Therefore, a room with pillows and mattresses offers the opportunity for a regression where the children can just disappear into the cushions.

With one of the regressive children we introduced a growing exercise. He was asked to lie on his side and curl up. The therapist put one of her hands at his head, the other under his feet, and gave him some resistance while he was asked to expand a little each time he breathed in. Regression is not so frightening for the child (and for the therapist) when they know ways to grow.

It is important to avoid total regressions but allow and encourage partial ones. The child is allowed to behave below his age and to be met on more infantile needs, but at the same time we want to keep part of his ego functioning according to his age. A boy can get a foot massage, but we ask him to sit up instead of lying down. A girl is curling up in the cushions, but we tell her to stay in contact with the therapist. After a couple of minutes we ask her to stand on her feet.

Nurturing Exercises

Maybe these should not be called 'exercises' because they include procedures like covering the child with a blanket, giving gentle massage, and so forth, which increase the children's ability to be receptive and to feel pleasure. This can be extremely difficult for abused and insecure children. One abused little girl said: 'Maybe you will suddenly touch my private parts. I know you won't, but I can't help thinking of it.'

Cooperative Exercises

Here we help the children use their bodies together with the therapist. For example: child and therapist are lying on their backs, feet against each other and bicycling. Sometimes the therapist determines the speed and direction, sometimes the child does it. 'Row your boat' and other children's games can be very useful.

Distance Exercises

Here we let the child and/or the therapist move in the room. What kind of distance or closeness feels good? When is it too overwhelmingly close? When does the feeling of being abandoned arise? Can the child ask the therapist to come closer or to move away? Can the child move to a distance where he feels comfortable? It is often difficult to feel what is good and more so to express it openly.

Sitting side by side, separate but close, is yet another option. This can give the child the experience of having an adult on his side.

Using the Exercises

There are considerations concerning the use of the exercises before, during, and after the sessions.

Before the Session

The sessions always consist of a well-defined programme of one to four exercises that the child knows. The programme is often based upon an agreement between child and therapist. New exercises are suggested and explained by the therapist before they are carried out.

During the Session

The children are seldom pushed to do exercises, but for children with low self-confidence who usually say no to everything, one may use mild pressure and persuasion.

Sometimes, strong feelings come up. The therapists needs all his skill and experience to manage such situations. Sometimes the sessions must be limited to 10–15 min to be manageable. Sometimes it is necessary to break off the programme and just talk.

After the Session

It is very important to process the exercises after the sessions. The therapist and the child talk about the different exercises and what they experienced. The therapist takes notes from these evaluations, not only for supervision, but to use with the child before the next body therapy session. This gives the child a feeling of importance, of continuity, and of control over the modification of the exercise programme.

Clinical Examples

Robert was 7 years old when he came to our unit. He stayed for 3 years and had individual bioenergetic sessions for 2 years.

At the age of 1 year he was moved to his foster home from an orphanage where he had been for some months because his parents had severely neglected him. We know little about his life before the orphanage except that his father had sexually abused Robert's older brother and had probably abused Robert also. A year after he came to his foster home, the foster mother gave birth to a boy. When Robert was 3, the family accepted his 5-year-old brother as a foster child also. Robert was referred to us by his kindergarten teacher because of a seemingly total arrest in his social and intellectual development. He was sitting silent in a corner all the time. When he came to us it was revealed that his older brother had sexually abused him and threatened to kill him if he told the foster parents, who had managed to be unaware of this abuse. The older brother was moved to another foster home. It later became clear that Robert also abused his younger brother, which means that Robert was both a victim and an offender.

Robert was extremely fragile and scared when he came to us. His anxiety easily mounted to panic with uncontrolled aggressive acting out. At other times he regressed, hiding himself in a corner, with his thumb in his mouth. One big difficulty was that every emotion was immediately sexualised. Joy, sadness, anger – everything gave him erections – which he could verbalise: 'I only feel it in my penis'. Often when an adult tried to be kind, read to him, or sit and play with him, he began sexual movements. He quickly provoked sexual behaviour with the other children at the clinic, and it was easy for the adults to get angry at him. How were we to work bodily with this boy? His milieu therapist was an experienced and devoted psychiatric nurse who also attended bioenergetic exercise classes.

Just being inside our 'cushion room' invited him to regress, jumping into the cushions, hiding, and sucking his thumb. We started with simple grounding exercises, standing up and lying down. He was restless, moving before he could feel. Lying down scared him. He jumped up and ran into the cushions.

We introduced the growing exercise described above. He enjoyed this. Supporting his feet in growing made him able to stand on his feet for some time. He said with some surprise: 'I can feel something going from my feet to my head.' He started to pay attention to his breathing and reported that breathing made his feeling stronger.

We also worked with Robert in a sitting position, the therapist holding his feet, gently pressing them on the floor to support his grounding. After some time he could go from a sitting to a standing position. He also began to enjoy lying down. 'You know, this is better than standing', he said. Being more grounded allowed him to start talking about his brother's abuse.

At first he said that he enjoyed his brother's sexual and sadistic 'play', but gradually he admitted that he was angry and dared to express it.

As a child whose boundaries had not been respected, it was important to start with boundary exercises. He was encouraged to divide the room with pillows and blankets. He would walk along the border of 'his' room, tramping his feet on the floor, shouting 'No'! Suddenly, he would fall down, as if all energy were lost. He became sad and then regressed. He then was encouraged to creep on his hands and knees. He could manage this. Slowly, he would regain the strength in his feet and come up again.

There was no constant progress in the therapy. An exercise that one day could give him joy and a feeling of strength could the next week arouse a feeling of catastrophe. He would shout: 'Blood! Death! Collision!' He talked a lot about his bad dreams, and about his brother. Sometimes he did not want to do any exercises. This was respected as a sign of his growing ability to feel what was good for him.

Sexual movements came up from time to time during the exercises. He asked his therapist if she liked him and loved him. When she said 'yes', he asked why she would not have sex with him. She explained to him the difference between children and adults. She assured him that when he grew up he could meet a girl and have sex with her, but now he needed to be a child and be treated like a child.

More and more he was able to express his feeling of joy, strength, anger, and sadness. He would say: 'Can you see I am as strong as steel? I was so weak before and now I am strong. Can you see it?' He made a remarkable statement. He said: 'I was born ten years ago, but I have not lived for ten years.'

His body and his way of moving have changed a lot and so has the expression in his face and in his eyes. He has started to learn at school. After being with us for 2 years, he told us that he would never leave the clinic, but after 3 years, he was proud of being able to go to a 'real school'. He is also starting to identify with his rather sporty foster father. He will continue with individual psychotherapy on an out-patient basis for some time.

Alice was referred to our in-patient unit from her school at the age of 7 and she stayed with us for nearly 2 years. When she came, she was hiding herself, pulling her sweater over her head, sucking her thumb, and always letting other children go before her. She and her 2 younger siblings were living with their mother who was warm and devoted but immature and not able to take proper care of her children. The mother had divorced the father some years before. He was unemployed, drug addicted, and had sexually abused the 2 daughters. When Alice was with us, he finally admitted his abuse. This was a great relief for Alice, who until then had felt guilty for the breakdown of the family.

Alice is a thin girl who seems almost transparent. Her attitudes and behaviour rapidly change from being warm and affectionate to clinging and demanding or to rejecting and hostile. Sometimes she is a grownup who takes care of the family (like her mother wants her to). Sometimes she is a baby, and sometimes a premature sexually seducing teenage girl provoking the boys at our clinic. She splits adults into some good ones and some bad ones.

She immediately liked the body therapy and had better contact with her body than we imagined. We started with distance exercises. She was able to report what kind of distance was good for her.

She could report that when she was on hands and knees, she was strong in her shoulders and upper body, but weak in her lower part. She loved the growing exercise. She insisted on being small for quite a while and decided herself when to grow.

We introduced an expressive exercise. She would lie on her back and kick away a pillow that the therapist held up. First, she refused. When the therapist asked if she knew why she would not do it, she said: 'Yes... and don't say it.' Obviously Alice understood that this exercise was connected to her father's abuse and her suppressed feelings towards him. In the next session she explicitly asked for this exercise and put a lot of energy and anger into it.

From time to time she would regress, sucking her fingers, or biting on all the mattresses and cushions in the room. When she was then offered a towel to bite on she said with a smile: 'Do you really mean that I can bite as much as I want?' She could feel the strength in her jaw and teeth while the therapist pulled the towel she was biting.

Slowly, she was able to accept and tolerate her strong feelings and to integrate and express them directly instead of repressing them or dissociating.

Chris was 9 years old when she came to our clinic and was an in-patient for 10 months. She was less disturbed than Robert or Alice. She was referred to us because of severe encopresis. She had repeated urinary infections and had been in and out of hospitals since she was 4 years old. Her first hospitalisation was when her brother, who later grew up to be the 'perfect' child in the family, was born. The parents had given up and rejected Chris. They experienced her encopresis as an aggressive act against them.

In the body therapy we started with hold and let go exercises. She was asked to hold her breath, to make fists, and to then let go. We then had the therapist hold her wrists so Chris could shout: 'Let me go! Get away!' We worked hard to help her feel and express her aggression. Slowly she was able to express more anger. Eventually, she could throw a pillow on the floor and say 'No!' One day she suddenly started shouting: 'Hell! Shit! Fuck!' This was a turning point and afterwards she was less tense.

An exercise of walking on her buttocks helped Chris feel more sensations in this part of her body. What continued to be difficult for her was accepting the therapists care, support, and soft massage. It was also difficult for her to ask for help.

Although her total situation improved, Chris was discharged before her problems were worked through. Nonetheless, the bioenergetic work was of great importance. Chris and her family were offered family therapy on an out-patient basis.

Discussion

At our clinic we evaluate our entire programme every 6 months. The milieu therapists find that the body therapy is an increasingly important part of our programme, but they also find this work difficult and demanding. They find too little time for preparation before and reflection after the sessions in our busy ward. As the therapists are divided into two groups, they only get supervision every 2nd week. I agree with them that this is not enough. It has been an exciting experience and a great challenge to all of us to develop this kind of bioenergetic work with children. This is a continuing process at the unit. The clear structure of the programme reduces regressive, sexualised, and aggressive behaviour to manageable levels without completely stopping such behaviour. It is obvious to all therapists and team workers at our clinic that the children benefit greatly from this body therapy, and the children usually are very eager to have the sessions. This enthusiasm gives us energy and courage to go on with the work.

In my own view it is not only the children who benefit from the introduction of bioenergetic work. The milieu therapists are provided with a setting where attachment and relationships can grow. And their understanding of the general psychodynamics of the children has greatly improved. The bioenergetic approach increases their ability to use their eyes as an important instrument for understanding. Their ability to tolerate and handle strong emotions has also improved outside the body therapy sessions.

My conclusions are:

Properly designed bioenergetic exercises have proven useful in body therapy with children. Children respond surprisingly well to these concrete, bodily approaches. (Perhaps we should not be surprised since bodily expressions are much closer to children than to the more verbal adults.)

Our modification of bioenergetic therapy can be carried out by experienced milieu therapists if they are supervised by bioenergetic therapists.

Ego-building bioenergetic therapy can be used successfully with severely disturbed children. It can contribute to the building of therapeutic relationships, to the development of attachment, and to the growth of the ego.

Some of the principles from our work with disturbed children may be also valuable in working with adults with borderline, narcissistic, and schizoid character disorders.

Based on our experience, it is possible to develop an individual child psychotherapy based on bioenergetic analysis.

My hopes are:

That we collect the present knowledge and experience of bioenergetic therapists who have worked with children and adolescents; that we continue to develop bioenergetic therapy for children and put more energy into further investigations and explorations, and that bioenergetic child analysis will be a substantial part of the International Institute for Bioenergetic Analysis in the future.

References

Bowlby J (1988) A Secure Base. Routledge, London.
Helfaer PM (1988/89) The hated child: An aspect of the borderline personality. Bioenerget Anal 3:24–44.
Lewis R (1976) Bioenergetics and early ego development. Energy Character 7(2):2–14.
Lewis R (1986) Getting the head to really sit on ones shoulder. A first step in grounding the false self. Bioenerget Anal 2:56–77.
Lowen A (1975) Bioenergetics. Simon & Schuster, New York.
Lowen A (1989) Some observations on the relation between the ego, character and sexuality, unpublished manuscript.
Ludwig M (1990) Swimming in a human sea: A developmental approach to grounding. Energy Character 21:62.
Sharaf M (1983) Fury on Earth: A Biography of Wilhelm Reich. St. Martin's Press, New York.
Waal N (1958) On Wilhelm Reich. In Wilhelm Reich Memorial Volume. Ritter Press, Nottingham (reprinted in 1973: Boadella D: Wilhelm Reich: The Evolution of his Work. Vision Press, London).

This article was reprinted from The Journal of the International Institute for Bioenergetic Analysis, vol. 5, no. 1, 30–44 by kind permission of Nina Halsen.

Halsen, Arnt Vilhelm, MD (1936, died in 1996), was married, 2 children. He became Chief of the Child Psychiatric Clinic in Fredrikstad, where he did psychotherapy with children and supervised the staff. He started in character-analytical vegetotherapy (Reich) and later (1982) became a certified bioenergetic therapist. He worked with adults and with children, being interested in a psychodynamic therapy. He has published 10 articles on various psychotherapeutical issues and in 1975 a book called 'Behandlingshverdag' (which translates into something like 'The everyday confrontations in child psychiatry'). His bioenergetic work with children did not receive the recognition it deserved during his lifetime.

Ventling CD (ed): Childhood Psychotherapy. A Bioenergetic Approach.
Basel, Karger, 2001, pp 53–69

Douglas, or the Paralysing Effect of Sensory Overstimulation

Suzanne B. Robert-Ouvray

Introduction

Psychotherapy with children under the age of 11 or 12 inevitably makes use of the body in movement or the movement of one or several figurines. As up to this age, children have a very limited capacity for introspection and for verbalising sensations. However, through playing, drawing and sculpting the child can express his entire internal world, often very clearly. A therapist must be able to identify with his or her young patient and to rediscover his or her own internal child in order to participate in the child's games, in order to help the child explore his fears and to allow him to integrate certain traumatic experiences left in abeyance in his psychophysical universe. Bioenergetics can be integrated into a child's psychotherapeutic process, but with some reservations. The positions of stress or tension encouraged in bioenergetics are based on the Freudian idea that the subject develops through frustration. I personally think that human beings develop through a dialectic between 'hard' and 'soft', difficult and gentle, tension and relaxation, that is frustration and satisfaction [Robert-Ouvray, 1997, p. 34]. Thus, a therapist can propose to children exercises that are 'hard' and distressing and others that are 'soft' and calming. Mentally ill children often experience major difficulties accessing ambivalence, which only becomes possible with the integration of polarities, be they tonic, sensory, affective or representative [Robert-Ouvray, 1997, p. 71–79].

Moreover, positions of stress are positions of bodily and emotional disorganisation and they test the subject's ability to de-structure and then to restructure himself. However, prior to the age of 11, which corresponds to the age at which a person integrates a normal motivity including a representation of himself with meaning, one cannot take the risk of de-structuring a child without knowing that child's ability to verbalise his body and his fantasies. In my clinical experience, young patients have demonstrated that there is no distance between their psychic defence systems and their psychomotor structure. Thus, in order to protect themselves or to defend themselves from others, they use the material of their own structure to project themselves onto the other [Robert-Ouvray, 1996, p. 67–68]. One must, therefore, be very careful with a child before having him face the test of bodily hypertension. One must take into consideration the psychomotor development of the child.

Lowen [1988] explains that bioenergetics comprises manipulations that aim at relaxation and specific exercises that aim at becoming aware of one's own tensions. I think that one can also offer children exercises which allow them to experience gentleness and relaxation, along with tactile manipulations that will give them access to 'hard' feelings which are very distressing for children in this age range. I would also like to specify that I never propose any exercise of tension or relaxation as long as the child has not brought me there himself in the unfolding of his story. Thus, I have accompanied children in therapy sometimes without the use of any psychophysical exercise.

Douglas

Douglas was nearly 5 years old when I met him for the first time. He was a little red-haired boy with green eyes. He did not respond when I greeted him, did not look me in the eyes and did not seek contact. He had been followed by a speech therapist since the age of 3 due to major language difficulties. This speech therapist sent him to me because she was not making any progress with him. At school, his teacher complained of his lack of concentration: 'Douglas is always somewhere else, on the moon; he never listens to anything; he never follows instructions; he is always responding off the point; he never plays with the other children; he can't fit into the group; nobody understands what he says; he's strange.'

Douglas had many ear infections during the first 2 years of his life. His mother spoke loudly, quickly and a lot; she trivialised and generalised all of her child's behaviour patterns. She understood and interpreted his mental universe with very simple, basic equations: He only plays with toy cars because he is a boy; he only names objects with colours because he is sensitive; he does not answer when you call him because he is a dreamer; he does not follow instructions and gets enraged because he has a strong personality. She affirmed that she knew everything about him. Every description of the child led to a personal interpretation aimed at making the situation less alarming. However, the mother complained about her child's behaviour:

he is an angel or a demon; he is aggressive with her; he is not patient, jumps from one thing to another, can never concentrate on a game; he is adorable, but sometimes 'it's like he's crazy.' Only spankings or cold water on the face would calm him.

His mother alternated between being defensive and being seductive. Her body moved away or towards me, her face paled or blushed, she twisted her hands. I got the feeling that she was anxiety-ridden, certainly invaded by an immense sense of guilt, and ready to fall apart. She was in a feeling of all-powerfulness. Her words made me think that she often behaved paradoxically with Douglas. She did not touch him very often and even pushed him away. She was very often overcome by death anxieties that had overwhelmed her when she was pregnant with Douglas. She was currently 7 months pregnant and much afraid of losing the second child.

Douglas's mother left no room for the father to speak. He sat docile on the couch, like 'a big timid boy', affable looking, but he did not seek to express himself. He did not take care of his child, but would take Douglas in the car when he went shopping. He did not seem to be at all aware of his son's suffering. He trivialised the situation by saying that he recognised himself in his son, that he too had been in his own world.

While the parents spoke, Douglas grabbed onto the toy cars and pushed them around on the floor in a line. He did not respond when I spoke to him, neither through a change in bodily movements nor through changes of rhythm in his gestures. It was as if he did not hear.

In order to make things go more quickly, his mother systematically washed him, dressed him, undressed him, put on his shoes and fed him. In any case, she said, he did not obey and she was always obliged to scream and to hit him. When the mother described this, Douglas got up and went towards his father with two fingers of his right hand in his mouth and his left hand in his pants. I got the feeling he was very anxious. The father seemed to represent a person who provided him with a little protection from the mother's violent and excessive behaviour. The parents went on to describe their respective families which suffered a lot and were organised by behaviours of alcoholism, intrusion, and emotional capture and abandonment.

During this first appointment, I suggested free drawing and Douglas drew a thin, fragile circle with two sticks coming out, one from each side. Then he took a second sheet, drew another circle, two limbs, hair on the head, with traits inside which could have represented a mouth, a nose and eyes. I asked him to tell me about his drawings. He did not respond, turned the sheet over and drew a series of parallel lines. Then he babbled to such an extent I wondered if he was delirious. I had the impression he had made up a language of his own. I did not understand what he said, but his drawings told me: 'This is where I am: I am a person who is not very developed and another who is more developed, and between the two there is a path or parallel lines.'

The mother continually intervened. She translated what her son said, responded for him and interrupted her husband. She took up all the space. I had trouble ending the appointment because her anxiety overflowed into an invasive logorrhoea.

I felt disconcerted by this child. His symptoms led me to presume there was a retreat at a young age nearing a retreat into autism. He was in relational avoidance: his face was serious, the look in his eyes absent and peripheral, he sat loosely on the floor as if he had no spinal column, he did not respond to his name. His actions did not encourage further interaction. Yet he played with the cars quickly and nervously, and I had the feeling that he was mentally following a story. This reassured me. I thought that Douglas was a little boy who must have had to confront, from the day he was born, painful over-stimulation of two kinds. First, there was an excess of external stimulation from his mother's hitting and screaming, from being pushed around, and from the painful ear infections. The child also must have absorbed like a sponge all the maternal anxieties which are all painful stimulation for a baby. Secondly, an excess of internal stimulation from an absence of any release of tension because the mother, too centred on herself, entirely lacked empathy; she did not understand her little boy but projected on him her desires and fantasies. She could not manage to make sense of her child's emotions and she did not provide any relief through tenderness.

Moreover, the father did not fulfil his role of providing support to help Douglas grow up. He did not offer his vertebral column for the child to lean on. He did not incarnate the third party, intermediary position between the child and his mother. He was undoubtedly very infantile himself and little capable of counterbalancing the strength of this invasive woman.

Since his birth, Douglas had found himself in a situation of terrible sensory and emotional overload that he did not know how to name. He had no representations for what he had been experiencing. He was currently equipped with insulating defence systems which protected him from external over-stimulation but which, at the same time, did not allow him to communicate with the outside world. He must have been experiencing immense solitude in an armoured tonic envelope [Robert-Ouvray, 1997, p. 178]. As a first stage, I decided I would begin by helping this child lower the psychophysical tension – combined hypertonicity and anxiety – by allowing him to express the terror and the violence he must have stored up inside himself. As a result, he would have access to other dimensions of his sensory equipment and be able to explore the imaginary world in which he had taken refuge. I would help him name what he needed to return to earth, to anchor himself and to brave external reality. These were my hypotheses and ideas when I started out. I would see him once a week.

During the first session, Douglas calmly entered the room. He went straight to the toy cars. His mother wanted to come in as well, saying she would stay with him because he was going to be afraid. I reassured her and refused. I told Douglas what we were going to do together, presented the different games and toys and asked him what he wanted. I was surprised to hear him respond in a simple and direct manner. He wanted to play with the cars. It then occurred to me that his incomprehensible and disconcerting language was a protective system screening him from his too-invasive mother.

During several sessions, I watched the same scene without being able to join in the game because Douglas ignored me: the child made the cars fall off imagined cliffs nobody saw. Short clear sentences alternated with unintelligible jabber. He seemed to be saying that everything was going to break. He knocked two cars together and asked one, very precisely, 'You didn't break anything?' The other did not reply. He did not create characters per se but he was very gentle with, attentive to and concerned about the cars. He completely invested in the relationship with them as if they were living beings.

When I asked him to draw a person, he sat down in front of a piece of paper and said, 'I don't know how to draw a person'. His voice brimmed with depreciation and despair. For several sessions, the child reacted to any offer to draw, play with building blocks or sculpt as if it were an order and he stopped himself, depreciating himself. This negative sentiment was linked in part to his mother's hold over his bodily activities (e.g. eating, dressing and washing) which deprived him of access to his own bodily representations and his own capacity for action. It was also linked in part to the feelings of depreciation which invade all humans whose experiences are not recognised, reinforced, or understood by a parent. Faced with an overprotective and possessive mother, Douglas no longer had access to his capacity for creativity and for developing his own desires. He remained in a state of responding to primary, fundamental needs: he needed things right now or he cut himself off totally from the world. He had no tolerance for frustrations and was incapable of representing them.

This first part of his therapy was a period of discovery of objects and the environment. We would spend several sessions experimenting with the sensation of his hand on mine and vice versa when I drew for him. I accompanied him in his activities and I limited myself to reformulating his sentences and to amplifying his emotional experience. For example, when a car fell off the cliff, I said, 'Oh no, it fell. It must hurt', or 'That's terrible, it didn't see the edge of the cliff! It must have been very frightened'.

One day, after the nth reformulation of this kind, Douglas went towards the pieces of paper and drew zigzags in red and black. He said nothing more, but I knew at this point that he comprehended what I said to him. Something of the boredom and sensory anaesthesia was breaking down under the impact of the emerging emotions of anger and fear.

From this point on, Douglas watched me, he listened more attentively when I named what those incessantly falling cars could have been experiencing. I thought if he trusted me more, he could certainly express his violence without fearing that he would destroy himself or me. I therefore decided to intervene more actively in the session. I built a castle in blocks and put my car inside it. He took a car, entered the castle and demolished it while screaming, 'I had a nightmare'. He did not say anything else, but I understood that he was speaking about the beginning of his life, about his painful encounter with his anxiety-ridden mother, with the outside world and about the terror he must have felt.

I did not insist, because it was in the difference of attitudes between his parent and myself that something could be expressed. The fact of not reproducing the intrusive actions of the parent, which the child expected or was used to, provoked a double feeling of worry and relief. This emotional conflict provoked an anxiety which would then translate into the emergence of an emotion or into an enactment. Douglas then went to the drawing paper, traced two tracks of different colours and said firmly, 'This is not a doodle, it's a drawing'. He was asking me to understand him, not to depreciate him and not to judge him. I reassured him that I was listening attentively, affirming to him that I did not know everything about him and that he was free to express himself as he wished. So he took another sheet and drew a person and a vehicle, 'It's a chariot'. I considered that we had completed a first stage when Douglas symbolised what was happening between us on a therapeutic level. He accepted the holding I proposed [Winnicott, 1960]. We had been working together for 4 months.

From this moment on, Douglas put me to work for him. He asked me to construct garages, bridges, roads and toboggans with different wooden blocks. He then caused terrible accidents, spoke rapidly in gibberish, but then would say no more. I became his right-hand man. I tried to introduce ambulances and tow-trucks but he did not react to my offers of repair. I had to simply reconstruct it all in order for him to continue to enact his destructiveness. The repetition of these scenes led to his first identifications with me. At the end of one session, he looked at a car and wanted to take it home with him, saying simply, 'It's because I have the same, it's the same'. Remembering that these cars are animated for him and that he breathed life into them, I interpreted this sequence of events as manifesting the creation of a link between his home and my office, between him and me. He recognised some similitude between the two of us. Differentiation would come later. By opening up this possible space of fusion, he would then be able, provided he felt secure, to separate and to become autonomous.

It was at this time that I thought he formulated the existence of his true self (different from me) and his false self (the same as me). Winnicott [1965] writes that the false self becomes established upon the basis of identifications and that it is represented by an adapted social attitude. To have the same car, to be the same car is being the other, like the other, in the image of the other's desire.

In the session just prior to the summer holidays, I sensed he was nervous. He coloured a sheet of paper red and for the first time drew a castle, his Self. He then moved on to the building blocks, built and demolished a castle and with a brutal movement, threw a block into my face. I took his hands into mine, told him the rule of non-violence and asked him to express the same thing in words. 'Not happy', he said. His feeling of anger was most certainly linked to the abandonment he felt about the upcoming separation due to the holiday period. I reassured him, saying that I would think about him. And then he left. This second period was a period of transition. A bond of transfer was in place. Douglas could now re-live traumatic situations with me and experience them in a supportive relationship.

When I saw him again in September, he expressed himself with less confusion. He had eliminated many of the parasitic words. He again put me to work for him but with a very authoritarian, very parental tone of voice. I decided to partially oppose him and I refused certain things. He gave me a black car and asked me to build my house. He demolished it with a police car. I protested: 'You don't have the right! It's not fair!' I played out what he has never been able to express: revolt, a feeling of injustice, powerlessness, opposition to his intrusive mother who knows everything and runs his life. Each new emotional situation that emerged we repeated several times. Douglas could then express his need for safety. He drew several houses without roofs (toit, in French, pronounced 'twa') or windows and asked me to add them. He needed something protective, a roof but also a 'toi' – a 'you', also pronounced 'twa' – and an opening to the outside.

In order to better help him express his fears, I asked him what was in the sky above the house. He answered very quickly: an aeroplane, a helicopter and a vessel, but he did not want to draw them. Drawing them meant making them appear, and Douglas was feeling a lot of anxiety. With his agreement, I took his hand to draw the plane and the helicopter, but he did not want to draw the vessel. Then in one of the following sessions, he drew a red house around which there were other smaller houses, some orange, violet and blue, one yellow and one green. He declared, 'The yellow is a boy, the green a girl'. At this point I knew the yellow represented him and the green undoubtedly represented his little sister, born a few months earlier. Later he would draw a person and would write his first name in capital letters. It took us 1 year to attain a climate sufficiently safe for this, and for Douglas to feel ready to confront the enormous fears that paralysed him and kept him from existing fully.

During the first period of the second part of his therapy, Douglas expressed his archaic anxieties of being devoured. First, he drew a red witch eating a child. Then he spent several sessions drawing witches doing bad things and then tore up these drawings before throwing them away. I encouraged him to speak to the witch and tell her everything he held against her. He beat on cushions, fought with a big pillow, wrestled with a blanket. He always came out victorious and happy.

Slowly he came out of the paralysed state in which he had been tetanised [Robert-Ouvray, 1998, p. 41–43]. One day, Douglas sat a red and a yellow car down next to me and ordered me to enact a scene. 'Do it!' he said. I introduced a mean person who wanted to steal the red car. Douglas took up the yellow one and killed the thief. Then he announced that the red car just became the mother of the yellow car. I understood this as follows: if the mean mother disappeared (the character), the good mother could appear (red) for her child (yellow).

I said, 'This car (the yellow one) would like a mother who protects him from the bad people'.

'Yes', he responded.

He was able to conceive of a 'good mother' (a good object) who would protect him and defend him against the bad. But a difficulty arose: the child took out two other trucks, one yellow and one blue and spoke to my red car. 'I am your mother', he said making the yellow truck speak, 'Come with us!' His tone was authoritarian. (I think that the trucks represented the grandparents who were very possessive according to Douglas's mother.)

I, being the red car, his good mother, protested a little, 'No. I'm staying here. I am the mother of my child, I am no longer your little girl'.

He moved his yellow car away, 'No, I'm going with my parents', he replied, submissive. I felt very moved by this sequence of events. Douglas seemed in despair in telling me that his mother could not become a good mother as long as she remained subjected to and under the influence of her own parents.

He drew a witch and threw it away. He was getting rid of terrorising parental images and was cleaning up his fantasy world. When I suggested he should draw a fairy, he drew a daddy-fairy which he threw away quickly. The representations of his mother were split into good and bad, but he was in an emotional and representative ambivalence over his father. I then drew a 'whole' good fairy, that is, one representing full satisfaction, the ideal other. He watched, surprised, then took my pen, wrote his name, folded the paper, stapled it and took it home with him. I had become the good object upon which he could lean in order to exist. The therapeutic idea is to help the child counterbalance the presence of an internalised 'bad parent' with good elements – the 'bad parent' corresponding to the sensory-tonic state, not the person, at moments when the parent is not satisfying the child fully, and the 'good parent' being that state at times of satisfaction. The creating of a link and the dialectic between opposing poles allows the integration of these experiences [Robert-Ouvray, 1996, p. 94–102].

Then Douglas would move on to explore how the bad parent made him suffer: by denying his actions and his productions, by causing him fear through the fits of anger, by subjugating him without any explanations. I helped him enact both the authoritarian parent who terrorised the child and the frightened child who dared to rebel and to create opposition. That would allow him to express the interdictions he had internalised, notably the one forbidding him to open up to the outside world and to have different and autonomous thoughts. By acting out the wicked witch who humiliated, depreciated and broke the emotional flow which brings jubilation in creation, Douglas had access to meaning, expressing the parental words, feelings and injunctions that were paralysing him in his actions and in his words. He was no longer just a bad boy who did not obey and who only did bad things, but he recognised himself as a victim. He came out of the paralysed state which had accompanied massive depreciation.

This part of the therapy, which separated the aggressor from the aggressed, the bad parent from the suffering child, made it possible to do more in-depth identification work. Two weeks later, Douglas arrived and announced, 'Now, my name is John'. I was not really surprised that Douglas approached the question of his false self in this manner, but it is more frequent for children to give another name to a figurine. In a breathtaking identification amalgamation, the child went from a nice witch to a bad one, from Douglas to John. Then the characters stabilised and the theme of the prison kept coming back: the subjugated yellow car went to prison when ordered to do so by the witch, but then ran away at night when the world was sleeping. It was very repetitive, rapid and wearing. I proposed having someone nice enter the scene to defend him. After a few tries with characters who run away from the witch, he showed his two fingers of his right hand (those he had put in his mouth). The fingers delivered the cars and the wicked witch, furious, died and fell into a hole. He had invested the two fingers of his right hand with the power to console and the potential to save. He re-appropriated his body and his psychomotility. He invested his organism as a body representing him. He revitalised himself and the psychophysical work could take on another dimension.

The repetition of the prison and running away scenes began to wear on me. I felt tense and imprisoned. Based on these feelings, I responded, 'It's too hard. Garages are for cars, I want a house for people. Come on, let's go draw a house and build it.' He sketched a house with two windows, which still had bars on them, and we moved towards the large, lightweight, rectangular cushions that could serve as walls. I helped him build a house. He got into the house and asked me to use building blocks to build a garage next to it for the cars. He differentiated the hardness of the car-objects and the softness of the boy-humans. At the end of the session he knocked down the house, rolled on the cushions and cried out, 'It's all soft'. He laughed. He had the sensorial experience of the gentleness and the softness of relaxing. Acceding to this polarity of the soft would allow him, once it was sufficiently integrated, to set up an integration dialectic between the two poles and to create intermediary positions [Robert-Ouvray, 1998, p. 87–104].

He then decided we would be two Johns, two of the same. He invented the game of the mirror and I had to do the same thing he did, and in his car games the red became the yellow. We were two false selves who obeyed each other. Douglas had a lot of fun playing the one who obeyed and he made a caricature out of the one who commanded. He had been in therapy for 18 months. In playing his false self, Douglas could get rid of it and access his real self. This second part of his therapy led to a period with more emphasis on analysing his identity.

A third part of his therapeutic work began with his return from the summer holidays. At the first session, he sat on my couch and with a very affirmative voice said, 'Let's talk a bit. I had a dream and a nightmare'. He drew a head with teeth and a lateral form like an ear hanging from the right side. 'It's an A. I did it! This monster scared me'. Then he drew his nightmare: 'The ghost is on the moon. We're finished'. He drew with crayons and spoke really quickly. Then he turned away from the desk and went to the toys. I was stupefied by the symbolic clarity of these drawings and his words. His dream was to succeed in learning to write, his school phobia; his nightmare was that his real self did not exist on earth, ejected like a ghost to the moon [Robert-Ouvray, 1993, p. 177–180].

He started playing again. With a little pink car, Tessy, representing a good object, he fed the red car which was imprisoned by the witch. Tessy demolished the wicked witch's house, and then Douglas returned to the drawing and wrote on the bottom of the page John-Douglas. He had finally established an alliance between the two identities. He was not yet whole, but he was no longer totally split. After this point, his drawings were more spontaneous and contained several characters. He drew a lot in yellow which was his identifying colour. One day he began this way: 'We're going to play the witch who is mom'. I agreed, but suggested he draw a tree first. Relying on my intuition, I had thought that in order to confront this witch-mother, he needed a support or something to lean on. With a tree, my idea was to help him explore his grounding and to make him feel secure. He drew a tree with feet: 'It's a crossed out tree because it's ugly'. His tree symbolised his life force and his ability to exist autonomously which had not been recognised. He had been cut off (crossed out) from his identity as a boy, from his ability to speak for himself, as a subject. He was experiencing major narcissistic suffering. He was undoubtedly also talking about his father who had not been recognised in his role as a separating authority. Then he added ears to the tree: for the moment, I was the one who was listening, who supported him and who guided him. He could then analyse how his tonic envelope had been transformed into a tonic wall [Robert-Ouvray, 1993, p. 171–173].

'The car cannot turn into a little boy', he said.

'Yes,' I responded, 'I understand, the little boy turned into a car to be harder and faster in order to escape from the witch'. Faced with terrifying relational experiences, Douglas's tonic envelope had become tense and hardened. The child found himself surrounded by a tonic wall that was as hard as a shell. Douglas identified himself with this hard and rigid envelope resembling the body of a car. He grasped onto the outside object, the car, which corresponded in a tactile way to what he was experiencing inside, somewhat in the manner of autistic children [Tustin, 1992]. Psychically, the protective envelope hardened and led to an psychophysical anaesthesia. The tonic envelope became an armour which contained elements of his true self. In fantasies, the real self was ejected far away, put into orbit, while the false self was at the service of the suffering parent and hid the true self. Winnicott [1960] underlined that the function of the false self was to dissimulate and to protect the true self. Physically, the child called on his back muscles and rigidified. He threw his shoulders back, and it was as though he were uplifted by his tense trapezoids. His feet were not sufficiently anchored in the ground. The child then asked me to play a John who was protecting him from his tyrannical master. We inverted roles. He could then recuperate the natural functions of curiosity and openness to the outside which belonged to his real self.

He played out the scene of a black aeroplane and a white one going to fight against the witch. Douglas was feeling his power and validating his rebellion. He needed to re-appropriate his aggressiveness in order to put it to his service, particularly to reinvest his learning capacities. This session seemed important to me. Douglas re-established the sensory black/white polarity which allows the sensorial analysis of different life events [Robert-Ouvray, 1998, pp. 88–89]. He had let go of the subjective values of yellow and red to step back and analyse life based on sensory polarities more universal in the common integration process. Just as extreme suffering and extreme pleasure are the psychophysical limits of all human beings, black and white are the extremes which frame the sensorial field. We would then explore together hard and soft, the things black and disagreeably, followed by the things white and gentle. One day after these exercises, the child got dressed to leave and said, 'Say John'.

'Goodbye John.'

He went out the door and on the other side said, 'Now, it's Douglas'.

'Goodbye Douglas'. He knew he was bringing to me the part of him that was suffering, the false self, the part of him that sacrificed himself for his parent, the part that protected his real self. I felt a very strong emotion of tenderness and admiration for this little boy.

The third part of his therapy came to an end when he drew a tree surrounded by a brown bark. He had left behind his metallic enclosure. He had acquired an internal feeling of safety great enough to allow him to confront his terrors without breaking down and without the need for too rigid of an envelope. His tree, metaphor for his internal psychic axis and his bodily axis, took his place in the structuring of the representation of his motivitation and of his identity as a little boy.

During the fourth part of his therapy, Douglas went from despair to hope in successive phases. He expressed that his yellow car, 'cannot turn into a man because he's not strong enough'.

Then I spoke for him and demanded from the witch, 'My son is a car. I want him to be a little boy'.

He responded, 'No, not men, they don't have any purpose, cars are better, they fly everywhere'.

I insist, 'We do not need men, we are cars'. In addition to the difficulties of change Douglas was expressing, I felt the omnipresence of the possessive mother who refused to humanise her child and to concede a place to the father, agent of the laws of differentiation.

'I cannot become a little boy because the witch will catch me.' The little boy was playing out the refusal of the law and of limits: he refused to leave the office at the end of the session, touched objects he was not allowed to touch, escaped from his mother when she came to get him. When I proposed we change roles and to be the witch, he refused because he was afraid. He began to feel his fear and he was no longer only in his fantasy but in his actual feelings.

I participated in his extermination of humans. We danced together, we made music and I spoke on behalf of the possessive mother: 'I am stronger than the world. I am the master of the world. There is no human on this planet. Everyone must obey me and do as I say. Ha! Ha! I only want robots'. I also took on the mother's manner of speaking. Douglas knew those injunctions well: 'Yes, master, good, master'. He was both excited and afraid, in an emotional oscillation that rapidly modified his facial features.

A change of identity was taking form. He was making enormous progress in school, but reading remained a problem because he was still too afraid to allow the words and thoughts of others enter him. His aggressiveness took shape. He now drew spaceships with grey cannons and enacted a war, 'because there are extra terrestrials in this ship'. The return of Douglas's true self was becoming clearer. The symbolisation was becoming more and more important. Together we drew interlacing shapes and Douglas placed eyes in each of the closed loops. He was under high surveillance, persecuted by the eyes of the other who judged him. He escaped from the witch at night when she was sleeping like he escaped from harsh reality by dreaming.

He then expressed his mother's intrusion of his body. He was in a prison guarded by monsters. I asked for his freedom on his behalf. 'What is being free?' He asked on behalf of the monsters.

'It's being able to be different one from another without being afraid.'

Upon his request, we returned to the games of being at school, with blackened and crossed-out notebooks or with a nice and valorising teacher. Rules of life and organisation were taking shape. For the first time, Douglas expressed tenderness for me. Working on limits on several levels allowed him to differentiate tenderness from sexuality. He drew a black, poisonous apple. He was forbidden to eat it. He writes 'LA', the French feminine article, and crossed it out. 'It's forbidden,' he said. It seems he was expressing that what his mother was giving him was poisoned because it was intrusive, it did not respect his body, his space by obliging him to be how she wanted him to be. At the same time, this forbade any relation to the feminine, because the feminine he had experienced was dangerous. His mother was nourishing him with the black of anxiety and of possession. She washed and eroticised his body to excess. She still could not keep herself from doing it, she says, in order to go faster, despite my advice to stop this practice. She was not tender with him, but her touch was incestuous, she overpowered him. Douglas felt this sensory abuse for which he did not have the capacities for integration.

He drew a no-entry sign blocking the direction of the black apple and an arrow authorising access to a red apple. He was explaining how he was poisoned and imprisoned by his mother. I reformulated for him the right to belong to himself and the interdiction for anyone to take over for him. The next time, he wrote 'LE', the masculine article in French. Then he wanted to play the car and witch game. For the first time, John played with a police car that made the law. Douglas felt that his mother was outside the law through the various behavioural patterns she used to capture him. The witch (the therapist) looked into the empty prison in the morning and screamed with rage. The child broke out laughing. Then he said, 'I had a dream. I had a friend who saved me'. He had introjected a good object which could save him from the destructive witch. Reparation was finally possible. He had been in therapy for 2 years. Douglas had, in a certain manner, recuperated his true self. When his mother rang the bell, he burst out laughing, 'It's a big dog with a big nose who's there,' he says. I opened the door. 'Oh, the big monster', Douglas cried out laughing. His mother was very annoyed, totally unavailable for her son. She grabbed him by the arm and left quickly in a disquieting state of dispersion.

The activities and the creations of the child were now found in ambivalent territory. Douglas drew a Tyrannosaurus swallowing a goat, and said 'He swallows all the colours he likes'. All of Douglas's emotions, all the sensory expressions of his being, his entire emotional life had been swallowed by his anxiety-ridden mother. Then, for the first time, instead of submitting, brother-cars opposed the monsters who had come to get them. The problem of limits was still present. He blocked the tracks on which he was prisoner. He little by little recuperated his true self. Remember the two human figures at the beginning of the therapy and the parallel lines? These symbolised the distance between his true self and his false self.

His showed more growth when one day with two cars, one – yellow – being called 'I grew up' and the other – pink – being called 'Jack'. He drew spots of colour and granted them feelings: all the colours were nice except the black spot which was mean. His supportive process [Robert-Ouvray, 1993, pp. 71–83] finally went beyond the threshold of inborn physiological tonicity and sensation, managing to reach the level of affect and representation, for which one needs the words of others to give meaning.

I felt the joy of success. He drew a circle around all the colours: red, blue, yellow and black. He had reached the stage of ambivalence. But at the end of this so important session, his mother said, 'This is the last time we will see you. We are moving.' Then, seeing my shocked face, she said, 'You didn't know?' I remained dumbfounded for a few minutes and then got myself together again and explained that Douglas and I should spend a half an hour together to close off the structures and to say goodbye. She conceded to this. I felt and understood the dumbfounding effects such an unpredictable mother could have on the child. I thought about Douglas and I hoped that we had reached a stage in his psychomotor structuring that would allow him to stand up to a mother who was so neurotic.

Conclusions and Insights

The first part of the therapy centred on the experience of our encounter. Like a mother with her baby, in empathy, I echoed his emotional and verbal expressions by giving meaning to what he made the cars do. He put me to work for him without really recognising that I was someone separate from him. I experienced a great feeling of isolation like what he must have felt in his relationship with his absent parent or the parent lost in her own suffering. Then, towards the end of this period, I was torn between two feelings: I was bored when he played in front of me without seeing me. He was having me experience the solitude and emptiness he felt when he was without parental support. I wanted to lie down on the floor and move cars before my eyes in a repetitive and hypnotic manner. On the other hand, I felt on edge, as if this relational link were fragile and could break at any moment. Paradoxically, I felt a hypertonicity and a hypotonicity at the same time, signs of resistance and mechanical adaptation to maternal projections. Douglas had me enact a situation that was very precarious, an imminent danger, a little bit like those cliffs the trains and cars did not see and over which they fell. Douglas signalled a relational break by entering into his disquieting monologues: he spoke another language, his mother's. He took up parental injunctions, scolded a child, presented arguments. Everything was said in a rapid, cut-up voice, the words swallowed, the verbs before the subjects, the intonations often authoritarian. Sometimes the words followed one another in a neutral voice. I wanted to stop him. I could not think straight anymore. I was in a state of sensory over-stimulation [Robert-Ouvray, 1998, pp. 41–47]. I felt the fear which animated him. He had internalised his mother's logorrhoea. The cliffs over which he had the cars fall were a metaphor for these ruptures in emotional communication with his mother who was suddenly invaded by death anxiety. He had been dumbfounded by this maternal violence, rigidified in a hypertonicity that stopped his thought processes. On the other hand, he was no longer connected to her and he experienced the anxiety of falling into emptiness. He held onto his mother's words like onto a fragile thread. He no longer spoke in his name. It was because he was able to enact, with my support enveloping and holding him, disaster situations over and over again that he was able to express his need for protection.

The second part of his therapy consisted of a major effort of putting into place the elements of his mental life. The expression of his anxieties joined forces with the recognition of the therapist as a good object. The introjection of a good object allowed the emergence of the false self, subjugated and frightened. This was a very delicate period for me because I had to help the child accept every part of himself that appeared while helping him to differentiate between what belonged to him from what belonged to the internalised parent. At the beginning of life, the child is a mixture of identities: in the presence of a 'bad mother', he is both author and victim of his own suffering, just as he will be saviour and saved in the presence of a 'good mother'. When the good mother is present and warm, the child feels like a good subject; with the bad mother the child experiences himself as a bad subject.

Children who spend the better part of their lives in hypertonicity lose the possibility of experiencing relaxation. This loss of psychophysical suppleness allies with a deep guilt: the child is both victim and aggressor and he will seek to mend this other who is still a part of his non-differentiated self. Hypertonic children can no longer manage to integrate what is good about life. In day to day life, they will demand it in the form of endless cuddling, sweets and material satisfaction and in the intrapsychic world, this demand for the good will be linked to an ideal self that takes the form of magic, all-powerful characters.

The third part of Douglas's therapy aimed at the analysis of the false self and the development of the child's true self. Douglas explained under which constraints his false self had set itself up. He therefore accessed emotional ambivalence, which is a space of conflict between satisfactions and frustrations, between the good and the bad object. The ambivalence is accompanied by an envelope that is sufficiently flexible and protective, and a large part of therapeutic work aims at setting up limits and rules for interaction. I experienced tonic and emotional relief during this period because Douglas considered me really like a whole person apart. I was a valuable partner for him. I could help him and he was aware of it.

Finally, the fourth part of his therapy opened up to a work in constant bi-polarity. By creating links between opposing poles, the dialectic becomes possible. We worked on despair and rebellion, valorisation and depression, action and passivity. Douglas organised his aggressiveness and put it to the service of his school learning. Like in many other therapies, towards the end of the treatment, his development became more complex because the integration process occurs at all of a person's organisational levels. I was pleased with Douglas's development and the difficulty for me was to avoid using his successes to fulfil my own narcissistic needs.

This psychotherapy lasted about 2.5 years. We managed to restart a fundamental human process of psychomotor integration of sensory stimulation. Douglas could have completely shut himself up in his own world and no longer have access to the outside world. His parents did not have the mental or emotional means to help him develop harmoniously. Yet, despite their personal difficulties, they brought him to his therapy very regularly. The final separation was as brutal as the emotional ruptures that the child regularly experienced with his mother. However, considering the stage of ambivalence that Douglas had attained, we can surmise that he was able to link and create a dialectic between the good and the bad object and more efficiently manage his object relationships.

References

Lowen A, L (1988) Pratique de la Bio-Energie. Tchou, Paris.

Robert-Ouvray S (1993) Intégration motrice et développement psychique. Desclée de Brouwer, Paris (ed 2, 1997).

Robert-Ouvray S (1996) L'enfant tonique et sa mère. Desclée de Brouwer, Paris.

Robert-Ouvray S (1998) Enfant médusé, enfant abusé. Desclée de Brouwer, Paris.

Tustin F (1992) Autisme et protection. Seuil, Paris.

Winnicott DW (1960) Processus de maturation chez l'enfant. Payot, Paris.

Winnicott DW (1965) The Maturational Process and the Facilitating Environment. Hogarth Press, London (reprinted in 1995: Karnac Books).

Robert-Ouvray, Suzanne B. (1949), married, 3 children, holds a doctorate in clinical psychology from the University of Paris VII (1992) and as of 1998 a diploma in victimology from the University of Washington, D.C. Her training as a psychotherapist involved classical psychoanalysis as applied to children. She calls herself an emotional psychotherapist, as her main interests are the early links established in babies between motivity and the psyche. For the past 3 years she has focused on the pathogenicity of sensory over-stimulation in early childhood; over the years she has published more than 20 articles and three books on these subjects. She maintains teaching assignments in psychology at the Universities of Paris and Lyon. She lives in St. Maurice near Paris where she has a private practice.

Dr. Suzanne Robert-Ouvray, 19 rue des Epinettes, F–94410 St. Maurice (France)

Ventling CD (ed): Childhood Psychotherapy. A Bioenergetic Approach.
Basel, Karger, 2001, pp 70–82

Traumatised Children: A Challenge for the Bioenergetic Therapist

Rainer Mahr

Introduction

The suffering that children undergo as a result of a single or of a recurring traumatic experience has many facets. It is next to impossible to predict any one of them. What we see as therapists is the manifold modified expression of an earlier trauma: New events, new experiences are continuously layered over the original event, sometimes loosely, sometimes densely in order to protect the wound. Sometimes children adapt by suddenly modifying existing behaviour patterns and parents are startled. What the parents often do not know is that for the child this is the only way to survive. When traumatised children reach school age, often in confrontation with teachers and older or rougher classmates, the syndrome is again modified and gives rise to hitherto unseen behaviour patterns. Parents and teachers alike become desperate and eventually seek help. The challenge for the therapist is enormous: the child often resents being taken into therapy and he has neither interest nor understanding in whatever the therapist offers, at least in the beginning. The parents expect the therapist to heal the child. What is the meaning of healing when it comes to childhood trauma? The psychotherapist, regardless of his therapeutic background, is unknowing of the original trauma, and more often than not, so are the parents. Therefore, the therapist will begin with what is on the surface and visible: getting to know the child the way he is now, trying to gain his trust. This starts the balancing act of feeling what could be beneficial, what would bring a child out of his protective armouring and when to do which intervention.

Even if we agree that the traumatising experiences vary greatly from child to child, they all have one thing in common: each and every one of these children goes through a dreadful, terrifying and painful experience which marks and hinders the further development of the child. The resulting type of pathological behaviour or syndrome varies and depends on the character structure of the child, but not only. The environment has an impact also. Thus, a child growing up in a surrounding where he alone suffers from continuous economic and emotional deprivation while everybody else has everything in abundance, will react differently from a child living in a depressing, economically and emotionally poor world where everybody suffers. Or a child could be catapulted out of a previously safe and happy situation, by a sudden trauma such as an accident, hospitalisation, anaesthesia, a life-threatening disease, sexual and other abuse, separation from a parent, death of a sibling or of a parent. There is a long list.

To question and reflect the traumatising structure of life-threatening events – the shock trauma – is of special significance to the theory and practice of bioenergetics, for this determines the type of body intervention to be used and if necessary modified to fit the situation and the person.

Theory of Shock Trauma

The ongoing theory about shock trauma argues that the actual traumatising event is not the prime issue. Much more relevant is the issue of the inability of the child or adult to leave the scene of the trauma, to flee for shelter, to fight off an aggressor, and this because he is either too small, too weak, too unknowing, or physically unable. Normally, the organism mobilises all available energy for fleeing or fighting the enemy, in order to survive. But here the person is unable to do so and becomes helpless. A child, in contrast to an adult, is rarely able to fight or to flee. Consequently, the energies mobilised for survival 'freeze', remain in the body. It is thought that this occurs in the autonomous nervous system which controls the fundamental functions of the living organism. Cognitive and emotional control systems have no access here and, therefore, cognitive and emotional therapy procedures rarely succeed. Body intervention procedures on the other hand, which lead to a reduction of the stored-up energy, have increasingly proved to be successful.

Bentzen et al. [1989], Jörgensen [1992], Levine [1990, 1997], Rothschild [1993] and van der Kolk [1994] have worked with shock trauma patients. Their aim is to re-establish the autonomous nervous system which was modified during the traumatisation. This approach makes sense. It also challenges the bioenergetic therapist. To bring the patient to verbalise details of the situation will make him re-live the situation and remember the threat or pain or hurt, but it will not change his body physiology yet. Bioenergetic exercises, especially the cathartic ones, may well lead to the expression of certain feelings, but if out of the context, are not producing vital changes in body physiology. The bioenergetic exercises must therefore be modified in such a way that they bring about a feeling for the muscular power or strength which originally was missing in order to fight off a traumatising situation.

Jörgensen [1992] and Levine [1990] for example ask their shock trauma patient to bring a person of great trust into the therapy session. While working with the patient and witnessing the gradually emerging memory of the horrible event taking shape, Jörgensen would encourage the patient to go to the person of trust if the situation becomes unbearable. Bentzen [Bentzen et al., 1989] explores with her patients secure places by asking 'Where to could you have fled?' The patient is lying on a mat and Bentzen lets him 'run' – e.g. make movements with the legs, similar to kicking. She makes sure that the movement is done with arms and legs in a co-ordinated way as in a real running-away situation. When the images of the traumatising event appear, the patient runs faster and faster, until he reaches the safe place.

It is not necessary and does not even make sense to go through the same routine with each patient, to do the same procedure in a ritualistic way. It is more important that the procedure is adapted to the specific trauma of the patient and that a truly safe place to run to can be found in his imagination. He can draw from his experience in real life, e.g. maybe the kitchen of his grandmother was such a safe place. For when he has reached this place and has successfully terminated the flight, his organism can relax as the danger is gone. We therapists can see this in the deep breathing or other body relaxation movements.

The theory about shock trauma emphasises that healing from shock trauma occurs by bringing the threatening moment back to life while at the *same* time and at the *same* moment feeling safe or strong. These two simultaneous emotional events create the setting for learning that today there is no need anymore to be afraid. It is all about learning to differentiate deep down in the organism.

Trying to bring together such a process successfully with children is often difficult. Children with shock trauma may not show the slightest interest in the offerings of their therapist. Perhaps the traumatising event is still too vivid, too close in their memory to allow to view it even within the safe distance of the therapeutic setting. Often a child is still dependent from the very same person who traumatised him. The security and comfort of the therapeutic setting is therefore of prime importance and an absolute prerequisite for the therapy. It calls for a high sensitivity on behalf of the therapist. He must be well grounded in his feelings to be able to judge at a moment's notice whether a child is able to go through the process or not and break off the session if necessary in order to allow more time and space to establish what was obviously missing before.

When all these very basic aspects of feeling secure within the therapeutic setting are respected and the patient can have the experience that today, years after the traumatising event, he is stronger, faster, socially more independent, then he will conclude that these dramatic events need not repeat themselves anymore.

The following two case histories will illustrate how these concepts were applied in the bioenergetic psychotherapy practice with children.

Dan: Threats to Life

Dan, 12 years old, came to our therapeutic centre because of fears so strong that repeatedly he could not go to school in the morning. His mother normally would bring him to school and collect him afterwards, but sometimes he needed picking up after only 2 h of school. There seemed to be no real reason for the situation at school that could explain this behaviour. Dan got along quite well with his schoolmates, his teachers cared about him and tried to help him with his difficulties. Since these fears disappeared in the afternoon when he could play outside close to where he lived, the suspicion emerged that Dan produced these fears on purpose because he was too lazy to go to school. Such explanations put children with school fears into a particularly bad situation. They are insulted, their desperate situation is not taken seriously and they remain alone with their misery.

Little was known of Dan's early childhood. The family had lived in Sarajewo, the capital of Bosnia and the father worked in Germany, spending only his vacation with his family, e.g. with Dan, his mother and grandmother. When the war in Sarajewo became increasingly threatening, the father brought the entire family, Dan, his mother and grandmother, to Germany. No one except the father knew the German language, however, within 2 years Dan spoke it perfectly. The mother spoke little German. Usually only the father showed up for parent-teacher discussions, demonstrating that he was the most reliable reference person in the family, that Dan especially liked him and that he felt particularly safe in his environment.

My first impression was that Dan's fears were the consequence of his war experiences in his homeland. Dan had been confronted there with the threat of cannon thunder moving nearer every day, had heard of the death of friends and acquaintances and had experienced the fear that continued to spread all around him daily.

The fact that his fears did not emerge until he was safe in Germany somehow makes sense. The human organism often permits the perception of fears only when the real threat is over. Beforehand there is no time or space, since all activities are aligned towards dealing with the threat. Dan remembers noticing his fears for the first time when he was in a department store with his father in the city of his new homeland. Suddenly he felt dizzy and experienced an emptiness in his head which brought on a panic attack, forcing the father to take him home immediately. These panic attacks re-occurred without recognisable correlation to his real situation. Some time later, the panic attacks in the school started.

At the beginning of therapy Dan's fears were so strong that his father needed to bring him. Since Dan still had large language deficits at that time, the father's role as an interpreter was very useful. These language problems forced me to try non-verbal therapy methods. I began with relaxation exercises, trying to invite Dan's imagination, guiding his attention towards inner images and encouraging him to follow whatever came up. If clients are able to follow their inner images successfully and can report them, a very clear doorway to the unconscious can be opened. As a therapist one can intervene very well, promoting certain tendencies, strengthening others or making alternative proposals - naturally always at the level of the obtained images. Dan reacted to this method very well and we worked quite successfully together for approximately 2 years. His images were always ones of large and small spaceships, which were threatened or which helped each other and defeated enemies. It became obvious that the father was the only person Dan could rely on. However, enormous fears emerged again and again about his father falling ill suddenly and losing him. The father was indeed overburdened, he suffered from high blood pressure, yet would hardly grant himself peace and relaxation. Since the family status was that of refugees in Germany, it was unclear how long they were to remain here and what would happen to them. This represented a serious lack of feeling of security.

The therapeutic work was intensified by the fact that Dan began to draw his inner images at home. However, it remained unclear why he developed such fears of school. Did he feel obligated to protect the family at home? Once the family was threatened by a drunk co-inhabitant of the house with a knife. Discussions about this event and the possible effect on Dan did not change anything.

Eventually Dan began to fantasise while on his way to school. He experienced large, black, threatening shapes that stood in his way. He needed to flee from them. Gradually he learned to grow stronger in front of these creatures, to get a grip on them and to trick them and control them. By and by he did not need to flee from them before school anymore – first in his own imagination and gradually in real life. He was able to remain in school on a continuing basis, his achievements improved and it became easier for him to overcome his fears of school. All of this was a very gradual and tiresome process with many set-backs and not a linear development, as it might appear from the above.

I had not heard from Dan for nearly 2 years when I received a call due to a substantial set-back. Everything was as bad as at the beginning of therapy. For weeks Dan could not go to school and he would wake up with fear and panic in the morning. Once again, there was no real reason for such fears. In the meantime, Dan had grown to be quite a tall and strong young man and he enjoyed playing basketball enthusiastically and intensively. His fears had arisen again after he had made a trip with his parents to a small neighbouring town. This town reminded him of another town in his old homeland. He said: 'It looked exactly the same ... and there on top of the mountain was the hospital where my tonsils were operated.' Then Dan remembered the terrible anaesthesia he had gone through when he was 6 years old. A mask had been put on his face and he felt himself lose control. He had wanted to resist and tear the mask from his head. But it did not work. His arms were held tight or bound to the bed. Helpless as he was, he had to surrender to what he did not know or understand.

It finally became clear after such a long time, that Dan must have been suffering from shock trauma. He had entered a situation in which his organism experienced an inability to defend himself, to flee or to find help and protection from a real threat. This had put the organism under such stress, that the organisation of the entire structure threatened to break down. All reactions around the fear, including the inner alarm system, remained alert. There was no solution for the threat that could signal relief and turn off all alarm bells. Since existential life processes had been threatened, the autonomous nervous system was affected as well. This is where traces of the catastrophe remained stored away.

Dan was now taller and stronger than he had been during the traumatising experience. Most important, he knew that he had become a fast and well-trained sportsman. His experience of himself was put in connection with the traumatising images: He was down on the mat trying to remember the hospital operating room. His agitation and arising fear were clearly visible. When he believed he could not tolerate the fear anymore, he began – as we had agreed upon beforehand – to use his fists to pound against the mattress to defend himself and to use his voice for support. After a while the tension dissipated, his breathing became fuller and he reconnected with his strength. The fears disappeared. In the following months this remained the course of our work together. His own experience of his physical strength, speed and power could convince his autonomous nervous system that the threat that had put his organism into a state of highest alarm was not there anymore. He could now adequately defend and protect himself.

Body work is not used in this context to help make contact with anger or other feelings or in order to reinstate traumatic scenes of the past. It is used to give the body a sense of size, strength, speed and agility with which it can protect itself from a threatening situation. With this awareness, peace and trust can re-enter the body, the apprehension of fear and panic may cease.

John: Games of Torture

John, a rather thin and frail-looking 12-year-old boy, was referred to us through his school, because of his frequent fainting attacks. These were thought to have a psychological origin and therefore I was asked to try therapy with him. John was considered to be mentally handicapped, possibly as a consequence of early brain damage. His ability to express his thoughts and feelings was strongly reduced, his verbal language was very indistinct and slurred. The level of his development corresponded to that of a 7-year-old child. John also suffered from a chronic cold. When he got excited, saliva ran from his mouth uncontrollably. His clothes were usually untidy and smelled like sweat. I always had the impression that he was highly neglected.

I became acquainted with his mother, who approved of the therapy, but seemed unable to contribute anything to illuminate John's history, nor to reflect or change her parental behaviour. She did not seem capable. The outer appearance and mental potential of mother and son often seemed alike. John had a brother, who, being older by 3 years, was superior to John and annoyed and tormented him over and over again. The father, dean of a school, never had time.

At the beginning of our work together, John's fainting attacks were the centre of attention, since clarifying this seemed to be the only interest expressed by the mother and the school. Due to the reputation of our specific work with physical symptoms, this also created quite some pressure on us. However, these symptoms could not be explored with John. He could only say if he had fainted or not within the last week. Since I was beginning to get the impression that these attacks could relate to inner tension, I began with passive relaxation exercises in my bioenergetic therapy room. I had him lie down, let him breathe deeper and tried to massage his chest muscles to deepen his breathing and to stabilise the irregular rhythm. I held his head in order to help him relax and make contact with him, which was rarely possible during a conversation.

This work showed no visible effect. It was also unclear if this kind of work meant anything to him. Moreover, after a few sessions, he brought along a few board games and invited me to play with him. Obviously, he had had enough of the 'senseless' breath work. He had to bring the games along himself, because in my therapy room there were none. He liked games like memory and checkers and he was so good, that he almost always won, which made him very happy, although he rarely understood how. I never voluntarily let him win. I tried again and again to talk to him, to ask him about the experiences of the past week, about his contact to his parents and brother. It became clear that the father was very ill and in hospital. John did not know anything about the type of illness his father had and was neither allowed into the hospital nor into his father's sick-room at home. When his father died, he told me this with tears in his eyes, but he could not express his grief in any other way. He simply continued to play.

Several weeks passed, nothing happened and we spent time playing board games when I grew rather impatient. I suggested we draw a picture together. I rolled out a large piece of paper, approximately 3 × 1 m, on the floor and laid out some thick magic marker pens as well. John immediately began to draw an alpine country scene with a train running through. It was an area where he repeatedly spent his holidays. He drew very carefully very thin lines in black colour, using only a very small portion of the paper. His inability to express himself spontaneously and emotionally were always my strongest impression of him. His very limited motion abilities were also very obvious by now. I considered joining him in drawing. I began by suggesting a huge storm coming down with loud thunder, flashes of lightning and pouring rain. The lightning flashed down on the train cars that John was drawing and rain poured onto the rooftops of his houses. I used my voice to imitate loud thunder. I interrupted my actions repeatedly to give him space and to observe him. First he tried to protect the mountains and especially his train from the storm by spreading out his arms over the picture. He seemed afraid and confused. Then he began to actively draw against the weather: he secured the roofs, drew protection areas and trenches for the rain water. As he drew he became louder and used more space on the paper, applying colour and moving faster and more aggressively. Finally, he began to use the entire piece of paper and allowed the storm to break out over the countryside.

I believe that through my invention of a storm, I stirred John up and enabled him to express feelings towards me: the need to give me shelter, to care for me, but also his aggressive desire to frustrate me. I did not wait quietly to see what picture John would draw next, nor did I admire his work, nor did I try to understand and to analyse it. I actively placed impulses and propelled certain reactions in him. Clearly, it was questionable whether these were reactive feelings elicited through my behaviour or if they were his true deeply felt self that became expressed. However, it seemed more important to me at this stage that he began to move, to expand, and to take up space for himself. I imagined that through experiencing his physical movements, he would be able to increase his feelings and gain a better sense of himself. Maybe, given permission to express his impulses, he was only imitating what he had learned from me and his behaviour would not be his own. However, every human being shows signs of imitation in the earliest stages of development. Distinct individual behaviour patterns do not develop until later through separation and distance.

This type of work was repeated over a period of several months, during the course of which villages appeared in the countryside and a few remote houses in the mountains that he visited regularly. Sometimes he would invite me into one of his houses. However, he would always let these visits fall short due to different circumstances.

Then one day John began to use material from the room which contained two huge mattresses, about 30 large pillows (measuring $1 \times 1 \times 0.2$ m) and 5 metal chairs. Thus, there was sufficient material to create various three-dimensional arrangements. John began to build the world that he had only drawn on paper until now with the material of the room. He built huge mountains and apartments for himself and for me, as well as discotheques, police cars, prisons and hospitals. I was invited into his houses in the mountains, driven there in a car (chair) and I received my own apartment from him that he either built or sold to me. Nevertheless, I was disappointed and frustrated each time: He could never be found in his apartment, our afternoon teatime was interrupted by a police raid or huge spiders would appear in my apartment, even though I hate spiders. Sometimes I was thrown out of my apartment, because it was to be torn down and I would end up out on the street. Criminals showed up each time who wanted to rob me and shoot me, or kidnap my friend John and kill him if I did not concede to their requests. I became desperate and repeatedly called for help by the police. The police would arrive, but always ended up being a gang of criminals in disguise.

For months the same scenes took place. The goal systematically seemed to be to disappoint me or to cause me distress. I protested against being treated and disappointed in this way. John would then calm me down and explain that the spiders in my cellar were not so dangerous and that the police would surely catch the criminals. My destroyed house always got fixed or I got a new one. Yet I found peace and tranquillity only for short periods of time. Then the torturous game would start anew. Even when I demanded to play something nicer, he only responded for short periods of time. No matter how much I refused to play, he always found a way to pursue his games. All attempts to find out who treated him in such a way failed. He pretended he did not know and continued to play.

During this phase of therapy John explored all his possibilities and as if to take revenge, to slip into the role of the great torturer. My protests, however, forced him to control his destructive impulses, though not for moral reasons, but rather to avoid losing me, his partner. He never gave in to me, but he did need to relate to me. He needed to include my needs and desires into his decisions and this meant that he was beginning to live in a relationship.

I mentioned that John also began to take care of my needs. I did not always want to fight or be prosecuted, I also wanted to go to a discotheque and dance. Only very rarely would he allow this and only for a short period of time. He would play taped music that he had brought along. Once I was even allowed to dance with him. However, this was obviously far too much and way too close. He never allowed this to happen again. He preferred the violent fights with the criminals, in which he played both the criminals and their persecutors where we got shot and hurt. If he was wounded, I had to rescue him in the role of a first-aid doctor. As soon as I had done this, I was persecuted again, shot or buried alive. All protests from my side did not help. Even if I played dead and tried to hinder his aggressive games in this way, he never gave up. He would give me so many life injections, that I was always revived and had to continue to fight. In his eyes a sadistic joy would light up when he would plan how he could ruin me in the next moment. I felt deep pain over the continuous abuse and it took a lot of energy for me to endure this. In the end I expressed my feelings loud and clear, I screamed and pleaded for help. (Even my colleagues in the room next door were touched by the despair that rang through the walls.) John was at times confused over how one could scream so loudly. Sometimes he would make a placating remark, at other times it seemed to satisfy him. In any case, he did not let himself be calmed or distracted by my laments for any longer period of time.

If I tried to take away a weapon (pillow) we would get into a tremendous physical dispute. We fought hard with each other, and I often ended up sitting on top of him. I realised that he could defend and protect himself but not very effectively. He seemed to like the wrestling and the body contact. He took every opportunity he could. I also encouraged these situations, for they allowed an immediate contact. For a brief period we would not be defined by our roles, but could be simply spontaneous. I was very glad for the physical contact, especially since contact on a verbal level was so difficult with him. He obviously was too, for he showed very clearly what he wanted and what not. I had no chance of pursuing anything he did not want. He showed me this every step of the way.

Another phase in the course of therapy began when John discovered our video camera. He wanted to install it in the therapy room and record our games. I agreed because I enjoy using the camera for children and adults as a means of getting in touch with their self image, using the feedback to strengthen their sense of identity. During the next few months, John always made sure that the camera was on, but he was never interested in watching the movie again. He obviously did not want to see himself, but wanted a witness for what was happening to him and to me during the sessions.

It became obvious to me that his individuation process was developing fast – independent of the therapy – when I began to get invited to his 'apartment' to watch sex videos. It was very important to him that we lie next to each other and that we get comfortable. However, I could not seem to find out what exactly happened in his movies. I would say to him occasionally that I thought it was a good idea to watch these movies and that it was much nicer than being tortured and killed all the time. But he never forgot to return to his old game of destroying lovely situations, of persecuting me and torturing me. His destructive tendency even increased when he started bringing women into the game. Sometimes we each had a woman (in the shape of a pillow) which we would fondle. Most of the time, however, he wanted to take my woman away from me, kidnap her and threaten me that he would shoot her. Then there were games in which I was a doctor in a hospital and he was my boss, having a good time with several women. It was most amusing to him to call me in for an emergency and then seduce my wife in the meantime. This would lead to consistent fights because obviously, I would not let him take my wife away. I told him to go find his own wife. The fights got very physical. We would tear the women from each other's arms and fight bitterly man to man. It was obvious that John was trying to work through his oedipal themes. This need not be further discussed. But in the physical arena the confrontation was almost real. It unfolded on its own when it became relevant; it was not instigated by me.

The further development of the game was unexpected. John continuously got so enraged that he not only began to shoot my wife but began to trample all over her. He would be completely besides himself as he stomped the pillows. I used all my strength to stop him from treating my wife this way. He could never tell me why he must treat women this way, what they had done to him that called for such a violent reaction. There were situations in which he treated all women like this. It seemed clear that there was unresolved hatred towards women. I actually only witnessed scenes in which he wanted to possess or destroy women.

He put me in a difficult situation: it seemed almost unbearable to have to tolerate scenes for months at a time during which I needed to decide between my life or the life of my wife. My distress was even greater when I lost all options to reflect or gain distance during our games. Everything would happen so directly and so fast that there was no protection whatsoever.

Therapeutic approaches always support the necessity of expressing one's feelings, regardless how negative or destructive they may be. However, with

John so brutal and direct as he was as a child, I had my doubts about the benefits of this approach. Would it not become necessary that I interfere in order to strengthen his control mechanisms? The reality aspect of the games solved the decision making process for me: a man could not just watch his wife get brutalised and do nothing about it. Of course I would scream and fight and jump up, grabbing the killer and the torturer, and try to save my wife. In fact, I would continue until I succeeded. I am convinced that this is how a man acts. John must and could understand that one could not just idly watch. With this, I was not telling him that his anger towards women was wrong, but that he needed to realise that men who were strong and loved their wives would not put up with this type of behaviour. My protests did not stop him from acting out his anger towards women. Over and over he would throw the women (pillows) onto the floor and trample all over them. All of my questions over why he hated women so much and what they had done to him or any attempts to clarify remained unanswered. Either he did not dare talk about it or he had no language for his experiences, which could have stemmed from a pre-verbal period of development. I felt very helpless and saw the senselessness of trying to stop him. But he got the space to express his hatred and maybe that was the most important thing.

John, for the time being, has ended the therapy. He started working in a supermarket. The original symptoms are no more. This shows me that his development has made good progress and that he is capable of adapting to the reality of life. He has finished school and is in a special preparation course for the working world. He will receive a diploma with which he can begin an apprenticeship. John found a former teacher with whom he spends some of his free time. His mother remarried and had a baby in the meantime. The new husband seems to be just as limited in his mental abilities as John and his mother. John, however, barely mentioned any of these facts in therapy. This is why I was glad to hear that John could relate to people outside of his family. I believe that he will grow up faster and gather new experiences this way.

Psychotherapy with children works best over play. This is the level on which they like to act, learn, work and express themselves. Their play is mainly dependent on activity, movement, physicality and imagination. The therapist in some way is always brought into the scene. Play therapy with children presumably is helpful for the healing process by allowing to 're-play' problems and traumatic experiences in a secure and trustworthy surrounding. This releases the stress that has been built up over a long period of time. Insights into the body can be gathered as such and must not be worked out by the mind. All these aspects are very important for bioenergetic therapy independent of how the therapist shapes his or her work.

There are many good ways to do bioenergetic work with children. Surely, the work is much more diverse than our concepts would have us believe. Mainly, we are looking for new ways to incorporate our intent, not our techniques into our interactive play with children. Our aim continues to promote the spontaneous and direct expression of all feelings and the discovery of the body as a part of ourselves that we may move and use.

References

Bentzen M, Jörgensen S, Marcher, L (1989) The Bodynamic Character Structure Model. Energy Character 20:1–17.

Jörgensen S (1992) Bodynamisch-Analytische Arbeit mit Schock und Post-Traumatischen Stress. Energie Character 5:116–132.

Jörgensen S, Levine, P (1991) Shock/Post Traumatic Stress: Symptoms and Causes. BODYnamic Institute Publication, Copenhagen.

Levine PA (1990) Der Körper als Heiler. Energie Character 2:22–43.

Levine PA (1997) Waking the Tiger: Healing Trauma. North Atlantic Books, Berkeley.

Rothschild B (1993) Ein Leitfaden zum Thema Schock. Energie Character 7: 26–32.

van der Kolk BA (1994) The Body Keeps the Score: Memory and the Evolving Psychobiology of Posttraumatic Stress. Harvard Rev Psychiatry 1: 253–265.

Mahr, Rainer (1942), married, holds University degrees in theology (1968) and educational sciences (1977). He has been active for many years in his private practice as a psychotherapist working mostly with problem children and acting as a child guidance counsellor. He completed his training as a bioenergetic therapist in 1988. His psychotherapeutic interests span and combine biology, physiology and hypotheses of modern physics. He is a creative and critical writer as well and has published several articles since 1991. They deal with a variety of subjects such as touching in bioenergetic analysis, energy aspects, identity, body psychotherapy between psychoanalysis and physics and others.

Rainer Mahr, Dreieichstrasse 29, D–63263 Neu-Isenburg (Germany)

About Bioenergetic Analysis and Therapy

The International Institute for Bioenergetic Analysis (IIBA) in New York was founded in 1956 for the purpose of promoting research and education in the fields of emotional and physical health. It seeks to develop an international community of practitioners who understand and affirm the integration of body and mind and the necessity of this integration for emotional and physical well-being. The focus of interest is on the biological energy processes involved in health and illness. Therapeutic techniques are being developed which combine the fundamental principles of psychoanalysis with direct work on the somatic level... a bio-analytic approach to the treatment of illness. The institute acts as headquarters to its affiliated membership organisations and offers training programmes for psychiatrists, psychoanalysts, psychologists, social workers and nurses. The teaching is done in coordination with national and local societies in Europe, New Zealand, North and South America. Nearly all European countries have at least one bioenergetic society who all offer training, supervision and workshops for further education and development. Presently there are 48 bioenergetic societies with over 1,600 members worldwide.

If you are interested in finding out more and you are living in the USA or South America, contact the IIBA at the following address:

International Institute for Bioenergetic Analysis, 144 East 36th Street,
Suite 1A, New York, NY 10016 (USA)
Tel. +1 212 532 7742, Fax +1 212 532 5331, E-Mail iibanet@aol.com
website http://www.bioenergetic-therapy.com

In Europe contact the Headquarters of the EFBAP (European Federation of Bioenergetic Analysis and Therapy:

EFBAP, President Dr. med. Regina Axt,
Adelheidstraat 14, NL–2595 ED Den Haag (The Netherlands)
Tel. +31 70 383 28 28, E-Mail axtmr@knmg.nl

About Body Psychotherapy in General

A number of body-oriented therapeutic schools and institutions other than Bioenergetics within Europe have joined in an association (EABP). The common underlying fundamental thinking is that the body is the whole person and there is a functional unity between mind and body. A wide variety of techniques are used on the body by the different institutions, involving touch, movement and breathing. The aim of the EABP among other is to promote the dialogue and the exchange of information among the members to further their intellectual, scientific, creative and special knowledge and practice through conferences and congresses. Some institutions offer training, supervision and supply addresses for individual therapy and group therapy.

More detailed information can be obtained through:

EABP, Secretariat, Avenue Krieg 7, CH-1208 Geneva (Switzerland)
or Courtney Young (Secretary)
E-Mail cyoung@findhorn.org
website http://www.eabp.org

Subject Index